Community Resilience

The Robert Wood Johnson Foundation Culture of Health Series
Series Editor, Alonzo L. Plough

Community Resilience

Equitable Practices for an Uncertain Future

EDITED BY ALONZO L. PLOUGH

OXFORD
UNIVERSITY PRESS

OXFORD
UNIVERSITY PRESS

Library of Congress Cataloging-in-Publication Data
Names: Plough, Alonzo L., author.
Title: Community resilience : equitable practices for an uncertain future / Alonzo L. Plough.
Description: New York, NY : Oxford University Press, [2021] |
Includes bibliographical references and index. |
Identifiers: LCCN 2020048683 (print) | LCCN 2020048684 (ebook) |
ISBN 9780197559383 (paperback) | ISBN 9780197559406 (epub) |
ISBN 9780197559413 (online)
Subjects: MESH: Resilience, Psychological | Community Health Services | Disasters |
Stress, Psychological | Social Environment | Public Health | United States
Classification: LCC RA790.55 (print) | LCC RA790.55 (ebook) | NLM WA 546
AA1 | DDC 362.2/2—dc23
LC record available at https://lccn.loc.gov/2020048683
LC ebook record available at https://lccn.loc.gov/2020048684

DOI: 10.1093/oso/9780197559383.001.0001

1 3 5 7 9 8 6 4 2

Printed by LSC Communications, United States of America

CONTENTS

SECTION IV   ANALYTICAL FRAMEWORKS
THAT DRIVE INNOVATION

Introduction

Harris County, Texas, the site of the Robert Wood Johnson Foundation's (RWJF's) fourth annual *Sharing Knowledge* conference in 2019, has been tested. Hurricane Harvey, the catastrophic storm that struck just over 18 months earlier, was one of the worst weather-related events ever faced by the city of Houston and its surrounding area, and the continuing impact of climate change suggests it will not be the last. The city's 2.3 million residents have also dealt with industrial accidents, borne the brunt of devastating floods, and provided refuge to people fleeing other disaster areas in the southern United States and to immigrants from around the world.

In short, Houston has been asked time and time again to be resilient—that is, to prove itself capable of preparing for, withstanding, and recovering from acute and chronic adversity and emerge stronger than ever.[1] The theme of *resilience*, a term that is used across disciplines and applied in various ways to describe physical infrastructure, individual psychology, or community response, echoes across this volume.

Resilience is about a set of assets that allow a person or place to recover when adversity hits. Just as we must address the inequitable distribution of stressors that often reflect poverty and racism, so too must we grow the assets that foster the capacity to cope with that stress. Whether it is vulnerability to environmental disasters or chronic poverty, we know that the confluence of the diverse factors that impact resilience are closely tied to health equity.

In its efforts to move forward, Houston has much to teach the rest of the world about both the barriers to resilience and what it takes to overcome them. The region's experiences made it an appropriate site for a conference built on the conviction that systemic inequities are an impediment to that. Unless everyone has a fair and just opportunity to be as healthy as possible—which is how RWJF defines health equity—the ability to handle immediate crises and long-term stressors remains out of reach.

Introduction In: *Community Resilience*. Edited by: Alonzo L. Plough, Oxford University Press (2021). © Robert Wood Johnson Foundation. DOI: 10.1093/oso/9780197559383.003.0001

Just one year after the *Sharing Knowledge* conference, the coronavirus pandemic has changed life in the United States and across the world. The pandemic has exposed the impact that systemic racism has on health disparities. While this has long been evident, a disaster of this scale presents challenges to understanding what resilience is. Black and Latino people have been significantly overrepresented among those hospitalized and among those who die from causes associated with COVID-19.[2] And the economic impact has been catastrophic for low-income families, resulting in huge job losses, an unprecedented demand on food banks, and widespread inability to pay for rent, utilities, or medical care.[3,4]

As RWJF CEO Richard Besser wrote in the *Washington Post* early in the outbreak, "The failures of public policy and imagination have been stalking us for years, creating haves and have-nots. . . . Our nation's predicament today is both tragic, because so many people will likely suffer, and maddening because it didn't have to be this way."[5]

The pattern that has emerged in this pandemic era reinforces RWJF's focus on health equity and redoubles our commitment to building a Culture of Health for everyone in this country. It is not possible to achieve health equity until, as a nation, we address poverty, discrimination, and their consequences, which include powerlessness, lack of access to good jobs with fair pay, biased policing, quality education and housing, safe environments, and health care. The consequences of long-standing racism and inequity appeared to be moving toward a genuine reckoning in the summer of 2020, when the streets overflowed with protests. The demonstrations were an immediate response to the televised murder of George Floyd, but they were also a wake-up call to address the urgent and long-ignored needs of many.

The *Sharing Knowledge* conference foreshadowed that sense of urgency. In panel discussions, Q&A sessions, audience comments, and the informal dialogue that is one of the most enriching parts of the event, we heard a lot about the social determinants of health and the political and social context that influences them. This volume, like the conference on which it is based, is not only candid about the grim news that is daily reality for far too many U.S. residents, but also captures the optimism we heard at the conference and lifts up innovative ideas about how to make progress toward a more equitable society. One consistent theme was that policies and programs need to be informed by the people they most affect. Unless we ask, "What is important to you?" and then listen to the answers, it is easy to make false assumptions and design responses that miss their target.

Conference presenters also challenged RWJF to be daring in how we talk about the distribution of power in our society. We are very willing to do so and have included "community power building" as a key strategy in our grantmaking and in our public voice. We are inspired by locally-grounded efforts taking place around the country, some of them described in this book, which are trying to right these historic and continuing wrongs.

Progress also depends on more inclusive discourse, one that pushes us from our separate corners so that we can meet in the middle and speak respectfully to one another. Both personal experiences and data alert us to the value of forging connections, but the rifts in American society, fueled by structural racism, fragmented media, false narratives, and the loss of community ties, present imposing barriers. To come together—across disciplines, ideologies, race and ethnicity, socioeconomic status, and the rural/urban divide—means honoring the vastly different backgrounds and knowledge that leaders, experts, practitioners, advocates, and local residents of every stripe bring to the table.

All of these ideas and insights bubble to the surface in this book, which is organized as follows:

Section I, "Shifting the Narrative," explores the idea that attitudes about equity and perceptions of who "deserves" empathy or support, and who does not, are captured in our stories. The language we use to describe the status of individuals and the structure of communities—*illegal alien* or *undocumented resident*, for example—has a lot to do with the funding we dedicate and the policies we craft to address a problem. Contributors warn against default narratives that interfere with equity building and share anecdotes that untangle complexity, generate empathy, promote activism, and make us laugh. Their stories humanize hardships, deconstruct stereotypes, and even help us see that purportedly opposing interpretations of a problem are perhaps not so different after all.

Section II, "Systemic Barriers to Resilience," insists that we consider the history, social conditions, and institutions that make it much harder for some populations to be resilient than others. A legacy of policy failures has left its mark—some, such as the demonization of opioid users that can be traced to anti-Chinese sentiment, were explicitly racist; others, such as the urban renewal projects that decimated neighborhoods, not only were promoted with lofty aims but also proved deeply damaging.

Against that backdrop, it is obvious that personal determination alone cannot solve the nation's challenges. By providing the backstory that may have led a girl into sex work or a young man into prison, by shedding light on long-standing patterns of redlining and discrimination that result in housing disparities, and by offering an intimate look at families torn apart by immigration laws, contributors to this section shine a light on the damage that can be done by public policy. By uncovering hidden stressors, they also undermine the nonsensical idea that "showing some grit" is all that is needed to become resilient.

Section III, "Reshaping the Conditions of Places Foster Resilience," offers hope that we can press the right levers to do things differently. Concrete action steps are essential—an adequate commitment of public and private sector resources, nuanced policies, strategic practice innovations, and test-and-learn evaluations are all components of the solution. Equally necessary are intentional conversations about power sharing and engagement strategies designed to reconnect communities and promote equity and justice.

Much inspiring work of this kind is underway, often advanced by unlikely partnerships. A health insurer is taking on the issue of loneliness, business leaders are getting involved in trauma-informed care for vulnerable children, and environmental activists are finding common ground with public health experts. As our host city of Houston knows all too well, the unprecedented demands of climate change are already upon us, and much of this section is devoted to the pursuit of environmental justice and the imperative of fostering community resilience in the face of natural disasters and human-driven environmental assaults.

Section IV, "Analytical Frameworks That Drive Innovation," looks at the programmatic and research design and analytic challenges we must meet to cultivate resilience and foster strong communities. Pioneering technologies and novel ways to collect digital data not only offer remarkable opportunities to learn in real time and across large populations, but also introduce ethical questions about what we collect, who we collect it from, and how we use the findings. Embracing the social determinants of health framework encourages us to be innovative in how we conduct the studies, assess well-being, and take action, but the emphasis on underlying conditions also complicates efforts to measure returns on health-related investments. While rigorous evidence always remains the foundation of action, we need to think broadly and boldly about new and more inclusive approaches to gathering it in order to inform equitable research.

A transdisciplinary approach is core to virtually every dimension of a Culture of Health, and the partnerships that have been forged in some of the initiatives presented in this book bear witness to its value. True collaboration means not only engaging representatives of many sectors but also accommodating their multiple and diverse understandings of where we have been and how we can move forward together. Building on the *Sharing Knowledge* conference, this volume offers a complex and enduring narrative about who we are as a nation and how we can equitably share this common space.

SECTION I

SHIFTING THE NARRATIVE

Narratives not only reflect lives and cultures, but also shape and inform them. Classic fables and bedtime stories, stirring novels and powerful nonfiction, plays and films that move or entertain, analytic news and journal articles, and in today's era, tweets and other social media, all influence a society's beliefs, priorities, and behaviors. Well-crafted narrative anchored in sound data is a powerful tool for pursuing equity, building community, and promoting resilience.

> *Narrative is the poetry that connects the numbers, the music to go with the math.*—Casey Seiler

The five chapters in this opening section give testament to both the music and the math, the stories and the data, as they resonate across race, place, class, and subject matter. With their insights and knowledge, the contributors suggest the paths forward for addressing the inequities explored throughout this book and for building a true Culture of Health.

In chapter 1, "The Storytellers," Kenya Barris, a Black television writer and producer, and Jose Antonio Vargas, a Pulitzer Prize-winning journalist without legal residency papers, weave together research findings and personal experiences to create thoughtful narratives about contemporary American life.

The chapter opens with a look inside *Black-ish*, Barris's popular television series focused on a Black family living in California. Characters and situations reflect the experiences of one family, but the storyline is common to many. The chapter continues with Vargas, opening with his arrival in the United States from the Philippines at age 12, unaware that he was undocumented. Long after learning the truth, he took a bold step to publicly share his life story, using it to share a more accurate narrative about immigrants in this country.

Chapter 2, "Data and Lived Experiences Both Inform Well-Being," introduces some often-overlooked perspectives about what matters most to people. After presenting findings about well-being from the field of economics, it takes a deeper dive into initiatives in the United States, Guatemala, and India. These examples reveal how community action can be combined with evidence to support public policies that promote a Culture of Health and health equity.

The contributors also help us understand that researchers and policymakers sometimes make assumptions about what matters most to people that are not fully informed. Listening to the experiences of people who have too often gone unheard shapes the questions we ask, gives meaning to data and creates a platform on which to build healthy communities.

Chapter 3, "A New Narrative on Gun Violence," delves into widely shared perspectives on gun violence muffled by inflammatory narratives that sow discord even on issues where none exists. The three contributors provide data about gun policies that enjoy the widespread backing of both Republicans and Democrats and among gun owners and non-owners alike. They offer a framework for elevating areas of common interest in ways that reshape the public narrative without infringing on personal beliefs.

Chapter 4, "Immigrants in America: Stories of Trauma and Resilience," provides an in-depth look at the issues that immigrant families, both those who are here legally and those without documentation, face every day. Through the lenses of health metrics and immigration enforcement, research reveals the anxiety that seeps into the daily lives of children and families. The story is not only one of despair, but also of resiliency: A comprehensive look at Houston shows that a humanitarian spin on im-migration can promote resiliency for the entire region.

Echoing themes of fear and isolation, chapter 5, "The Toxic Impact of Life Behind Bars," highlights the cruel irony that poor medical care, vio-lence, and inhumane design are too often the norm in jails and prisons, yet these are the only places where there is a constitutional right to health care. The damage to health and psychological well-being accrue not only to people who are incarcerated, but also to their families and communities. In a country that incarcerates a higher percentage of its population than any other, a chapter contributor who served more than 30 years in prison puts a grim face on the health consequences of spending time behind bars.

As this book goes to press, the United States and indeed the world are reeling from a pandemic of a scale not seen in a century and an insistent, widespread movement for social reforms that address deep-rooted racial inequity. The outcomes are unknown, the future uncertain. Many people are struggling for daily survival, with little energy or resources to think beyond the moment. Yet at such a time, the narratives we tell and the stories we share about both adversity and resilience may be more important than ever. This part of the book presents some ideas and perhaps offers some hope that we can craft a public narrative to bring us together as we move through the current crises and beyond.

The Storytellers

Kenya Barris, Creator of Black-ish and Other Media Productions

Jose Antonio Vargas, Founder, Define American

The stories a society chooses to tell, and the people who get to tell their stories, become the filters through which we understand the world. In today's often contentious environment, tweets and sound bites that agitate and inflame readily become more influential than stories anchored in data and designed to find common ground.

When public discourse is distorted, social institutions lose their capacity to foster well-being. Building policy on information that has been cherry-picked to advance a single perspective does not serve the broader social good, but instead leads people to conclude that their perspectives are not valued or even legitimate. When this happens, they can lose faith in our social and economic institutions.

That dismal trajectory is not inevitable, however. As the contributors to this chapter demonstrate, well-crafted narratives that are rooted in research can enlighten, entertain, and promote thoughtful conversation about delicate issues. By moving past clichés and assumptions and including voices that have historically been excluded from the conversation, they give us the tools to promote an innovative, inclusive framework in which to create well-being for all.

This opening chapter of the book shows us the power of stories to move the goalpost beyond vague hope and on to the kind of meaningful change that can build a Culture of Health. Kenya Barris's television comedy series, *Black-ish*, demonstrates how research-based findings can be embedded into mainstream entertainment media, enabling people to learn while they laugh.

Jose Antonio Vargas gives us an even more personal perspective when he describes his life as an undocumented resident. Vargas came to America as a young boy in 1993 to live with his grandparents, expecting his mother to follow shortly—she never did. The fear, deceit, and anguish that characterized his own

Kenya Barris and Jose Antonio Vargas, *The Storytellers* In: *Community Resilience*. Edited by: Alonzo L. Plough, Oxford University Press (2021). © Robert Wood Johnson Foundation. DOI: 10.1093/oso/9780197559383.003.0002 journey through school and into adulthood and a career as a journalist are part of a larger and often woefully misunderstood narrative.

Enlighten While Entertaining

Writer and producer Kenya Barris's award-winning television comedy series, *Black-ish* (renewed for a seventh season by ABC on May 21, 2020), portrays an upper-middle-class Black family—ad-agency executive Dre Johnson; anesthesiologist Rainbow, Dre's wife; and their five children—as they navigate personal problems and societal challenges. Funny, poignant, and entertaining episodes play out against a backdrop of contemporary social issues.

The Johnsons contend with the everyday demands of a busy, bustling family (sibling rivalry, interfering in-laws, nosy neighbors) while also facing the complexities inherent in being successful Black professionals raising their children in present-day California. Produced for mainstream audiences, *Black-ish* draws millions of viewers every week, who tune in not only to be entertained, but also to absorb the hard-hitting messages that are often embedded in the show's humor.

Basing Story on Lived Experience

Barris says that he seeks "to not just tell a story, but to tell the story through characters who are fully formed, who have people that they love and things that make them who they are. If you do that, and do it quickly and correctly, it's much easier to take people on a ride." On that ride, viewers may be exposed to uncomfortable or thorny situations that challenge their perspectives. But if they also connect with the characters, Barris believes, they are more likely to open their own minds to new ideas.

While fictional, the characters in *Black-ish* are rooted in real life. Barris uses his own family as the template for the Johnsons, which allows him to draw on his lived experience to inform his characters and plot. He tries to be as honest as he can in portraying family life. When a viewer who looks nothing like him or his family says, "Your family reminds me so much of mine," he knows the show has hit its mark. He believes that "in not running from the Blackness of my family and in trying to tell this true story, people have found themselves more in it than if I tried to tell some broad version of what a family should be. It is the specific version of family that speaks to so many people."

Seeing the "Other"

Barris emphasized the media's tremendous impact in shaping the ways in which we see the "other" (those we perceive as nothing like us) and cited the current divisive political climate as an obstacle to recognizing one another as part of the same human family. "It's not about being Democrat or Republican or whatever you are," stressed Barris, arguing that narrow partisanship needs to be set aside. "It's about being a person and living in humanity and doing what's right."

But it is naïve to ignore the sometimes-subtle disconnect that can underlie even close relationships between Blacks and Whites. Barris recalled how incredulous one of his closest friends, a White man, was when Barris said that he had never heard a song on a video that received two billion views; none of the other Black people in the office had heard the song either. That eye-opening moment reflected the reality that Blacks and Whites inhabit cultural worlds that often don't intersect, something they aren't always willing to acknowledge and may not even realize.

"We're afraid to embrace the notion that we grew up differently," Barris observed. "We live in this world where the media shapes the way we think about things so that we're afraid to ask each other questions." Telling a story that reflects two or more perspectives allows people to "listen to it a little bit easier."

We need to be open to exiting a conversation in a different way than we entered.—Kenya Barris

Grounding Messages With Evidence

Television shows should embed data into their storylines, Barris believes, rather than featuring only opinion-based arguments. In developing his own *Black-ish* scripts, he blends evidence from multiple sources so that no one can debunk his message as merely a point of view. "As a writer you're creating fiction, but at the same time I think that point of view becomes so much stronger when it's backed by research, and by foundations and organizations whose purpose is to give us this research," he says.

What Does This Look Like on the Screen?

Examples from two episodes of *Black-ish* illustrate how the show treats the topic of race. The first uses research evidence, and the second draws on Barris's lived experience:

- A Black staff member at Dre's agency mentions a study that found that rich young White males are much more likely to remain rich over time than rich young Black males, who are more likely to become poor.[1] The character lists possible causes for this disparity—"imbalanced incarceration rates, employment bias, and discriminatory housing policies, to name a few"—and comments that "it all stems from institutionalized racism" reaching back to slavery. The episode makes the point that even rich young Black men cannot take their "foot off the gas" or have any gaps in their resumes.

  A Black colleague's humorous, yet pointed, response: "I once took a morning off for a dental appointment. Didn't work for three years after that. The next time I did work, all my suits were out of fashion."

- A conversation with a close White friend about how often they each get their hair cut (Barris every week, the friend much less frequently) led to an episode on the relationship Black culture has with the barber shop. The conversation helped Barris understand, and subsequently convey to his audience, the importance to a young Black boy or man of the weekly visit with the barber, a dispenser of advice and a role model of sorts who always makes him look good.

Barris's stories offer insight into the resilience of people whose day-to-day lives remain tied to the legacy of slavery and hundreds of years of cruelty and discrimination. At times, they also acknowledge the reality that continuing trauma undermines personal and collective resilience.

While Barris writes about a Black family and uses examples drawn primarily from Black life on his show, his approach provides a template for entertainment media to deliver other messages through story. Themes related to education, the environment, economic inequality, and other influences on health equity and well-being can all be translated into scripts that are as engaging as they are informative.

Entertainment media has an epigenetic influence on health. I believe that the images the media shows us are incrementally changing who we are within our DNA—on a cellular level.—Kenya Barris

Dear America: Notes of an Undocumented Citizen

Jose Antonio Vargas also uses his own experience to tell a story of life in the United States, but it is an experience familiar to the millions of other people who lack legal papers.

"Mama had told me the plan: We were going to America. I would be going first, then she would follow in a few months, maybe a year at most." So opens Vargas's story of his journey to America in 1993, when he was 12 years old. He hasn't seen his mother since.

Moving alone to California was Vargas's first life-altering experience. Learning he was undocumented was the second. At age 16, application form and green card in hand, Vargas bicycled to the motor vehicle office to obtain his driver's permit. Examining his green card, the clerk "lowered her head, leaned over, and whispered, 'This is fake. Don't come back here again,'" Vargas writes.

Despite the burden of knowing "I was not supposed to be here," Vargas finished high school, earned a college degree, and embarked on a career in journalism. In 2008, he was part of a team of *Washington Post* reporters who received the Pulitzer Prize for News Reporting for their coverage of the 2007 shooting at the Virginia Polytechnic Institute and State University.

After living a life he characterizes as "lying, passing, and hiding," Vargas took a step that altered his fate for the third time. His article, "My Life as an Undocumented Immigrant," appeared in the magazine section of the *New York Times* in June 2011. With this disclosure, Vargas became a public face of undocumented immigrants in contemporary America.

I wanted to convey the feeling of homelessness and trauma, to convey the frame of mind that takes over when you are undocumented.—Jose Antonio Vargas

Vargas instantaneously became a subject of interest to the Department of Homeland Security and an in-demand guest on news shows from MSNBC to Fox News. Seizing an opportunity to leverage the spotlight and reframe public understanding of immigrants, Vargas founded Define American in 2011. The nonprofit organization is dedicated "to changing the way we think and talk about immigrants in America today," he said.

Why Can't You Just Get in Line?

The question Vargas is asked most frequently is why he doesn't join the queue to gain legal status in the United States. His answer speaks volumes about the uncertainty that people without legal documents must face: The queue doesn't exist.

There is no line. If there was a line, I would be in it.—Jose Antonio Vargas

People living in a culture that does not authorize their presence face an impenetrable wall of regulations and attitudes that stymie their ability to engage in civic life. Vargas does not know why he has not been deported and lives with the knowledge that at any moment he might be. No law offers him a viable road map to legal status or citizenship.

Yet like many immigrants sent to the United States as children, he knows no other home. "My grandmother is a naturalized American, although I am more culturally American than my grandmother, who speaks Tagalog and watches Filipino TV," notes Vargas, suggesting the sometimes random circumstances that allow one person to reside in the United States legally and deny that opportunity to someone else.

Immigrants without legal documentation risk arrest and deportation even as they engage in routine activities, such as taking a child to school. The choices for an unauthorized parent of a U.S.-born child are categorically terrible: abandon the child or take that child to a country that may be dangerous and is certainly unfamiliar. (For more about immigrants in the United States, see "Chapter 4: Immigrants in America: Stories of Trauma and Resilience").

The Stories That Shape Our Culture

Vargas aims to challenge popular beliefs about immigrants by correcting inaccuracies, introducing nuanced perspectives, and mainstreaming alternative narratives. Immigrant stories are stories about family, about what families do for each other, he believes. "As a journalist, I think narrative is the story that shapes our culture," he says. "This is a family narrative we have to cement into peoples' psyches."

Describing families as "illegal," Vargas says, advances negative and misleading perceptions. After monitoring the news media, he urged reporters not to use that pejorative language. Taking that admonishment to heart, the Associated Press announced in 2013 that it would no longer refer to people as "illegal" and would abandon the term *illegal immigrant*.

Another priority for Vargas and Define American is to use positive stories to connect people on a human scale. "I make a conscious effort to name every teacher and mentor who helped me out," Vargas says. "There is a whole host of people who make sure that we are okay, but you don't hear those stories."

Define American seeks to infuse immigrant stories in the entertainment media as well, recognizing its central role in shaping public opinion. The organization has consulted with 46 television shows helping them to integrate immigrant storylines into their programs, including an entire episode of *Grey's Anatomy* built around a story of an undocumented medical intern.

A Final Word

The storytellers featured in this chapter come from different backgrounds, but they share a unique ability to weave together broad evidence and personal experiences. Through compelling language and style, their stories connect individuals to larger forces shaping life in the United States today.

Stories like those that Barris and Vargas tell can give voice to people who are marginalized, whether because of race or ethnicity, immigration status or engagement with the judicial system, or economic circumstances. However the narratives are structured, whether the anecdotes shared are entertaining or jarring, lighthearted or profoundly disturbing, they offer compelling and vivid accounts to illustrate how so many people live in America today.

Data and Lived Experiences Both Inform Well-Being

Mallika Dutt, JD, Founder and Director, Inter-Connected, Founding President Emeritus, Breakthrough

Walter Flores, PhD, MCH, Executive Director, Center for the Study of Equity and Governance in Health Systems (CEGSS), Guatemala

Carol Graham, PhD, Leo Pasvolsky Senior Fellow, Brookings Institution

Julia E. Rusk, Chief of Civic Wellbeing, City of Santa Monica, California

While Kenya Barris and Jose Vargas are central figures in the narratives they explore (see "Chapter 1: The Storytellers"), the contributors to this chapter take a less personal approach to their use of data and life experience. As researchers and community organizers they blend science and story to dive deeper into the meaning—and measurement—of individual and community well-being and social change. Recognizing that the way in which we understand truth is ultimately subjective, their work reminds us that we need to draw on data from a plurality of sources in order to tell the fullest possible evidence-informed stories. Their work also suggests ways in which individuals and communities can engage both government officials and the public to build resilience and advance overall health and well-being.

All four contributors offer promising approaches to discovering what is most important to the communities they study or serve and describe models in which local people are able to initiate the changes they seek. Carol Graham of the Brookings Institution describes economic models designed to identify and understand what people value most in their lives. Julie E. Rusk describes

Mallika Dutt, Walter Flores, Carol Graham, and Julia E. Rusk, *Data and Lived Experiences Both Inform Well-Being*
In: *Community Resilience*. Edited by: Alonzo L. Plough, Oxford University Press (2021). © Robert Wood Johnson Foundation.
DOI: 10.1093/oso/9780197559383.003.0003

how the city she serves, Santa Monica, Calif., is measuring resident well-being rigorously and using the results to guide local policymaking and practices. From Guatemala, Walter Flores shows how the voices of Indigenous people can authenticate challenges and prompt a concrete government response. Finally, Mallika Dutt demonstrates how provocative public service announcements (PSAs) can change perceptions and narrative, using domestic violence in India as a case example.

Economic Models and Life Satisfaction

If it is unusual for a comedy series writer such as Barris to care deeply about evidence, it is perhaps just as unique for an economist to integrate emotions into her work. Yet the tools of that discipline offer a way to collect rich data about what people value most in their lives, tell a story about their shared concerns, and foster policies that reflect common values.

Returning to her native Peru as a young economist and continuing into her present post as a senior fellow at the Brookings Institution, Carol Graham has upended the classic underpinning of economic analysis in which consumption choices serve as proxies for what people most value. "That is not what our data were telling us," Graham insisted.

The data suggested, instead, that traditional economic factors paint at best an incomplete picture of people's lives. For example, Graham mentioned one study,[1] conducted in Peru from 1990 to 2000, that found that, despite the rapid economic growth of that period, "Over half of people coming out of poverty said they were not happy. And a lot of people whose income hadn't changed said they were doing well."

The same pattern emerged in survey analyses from other countries. "The findings were robust across people and places," Graham reported. Clearly, parts of peoples' stories were being overlooked by traditional models and in the policies derived from those models. Interest in measuring life satisfaction started to gain traction in mainstream economics, although "some brilliant economists resisted it," she noted with a touch of irony. The intent of the broadened approach was not to replace economic indicators, of course, but to add nuance, detail, and human scale to them.

Surveying Well-Being: Beyond Money

Economic models that incorporate well-being indicators offer a unified framework in which to talk about both economic processes and human experiences,

Graham believes. But rigor remains key. "We are not just running around asking people what makes them happy," she stressed. "Metrics underlie the narratives we develop." (The next section of this chapter describes concrete efforts in Santa Monica, Calif., to apply this principle.)

By applying her modeling approach to Gallup Poll surveys conducted in the United States and internationally from 2009 to 2017, Graham was able to measure the relative weight of financial and other well-being indicators. The Gallup Poll measures and tracks public attitudes about a host of political, social, and economic subjects.

While income was the highest ranked determinant of well-being, several other key factors emerged.[2] Starting with the most important, these were post-high school education; learned something yesterday; no health problems; freedom to choose what to do with one's life; believing that working hard will get one ahead; high school education; and living in an urban area versus a rural one.

Seeing those values reflected in hard numbers helps put the daily lives of individuals into a larger context. The interaction between income and life choices as a driver of well-being is especially important.

> *People with more means have the opportunity to choose the kind of lives they want to lead, and that results in higher levels of well-being. It does not mean more and more money makes you more and more happy.*—Carol Graham

Key factors associated with unhappiness and ill-being, starting with the one most strongly associated with unhappiness are: being between the ages of 45 and 54 (rather than between ages 15 and 24, 25 and 44, or over 54); being unemployed versus being employed full time; being divorced or separated compared to being married.

The association between age and ill-being indicates that happiness and life satisfaction are U-shaped—happiness decreases into middle age and increases as people age, so long as they are healthy. "As people get older, aspiration aligns with reality, and they get happier," Graham said. She also noted a selection bias in that happier people tend to live longer than less happy people.

The finding that being divorced or separated is associated with ill-being should not be interpreted to suggest the reverse is true—that being married per se has a lasting effect on well-being, Graham cautioned. No evidence of a positive effect was found in societies in which people marry because they feel pressed to conform to social norms that place high value on marital status. Selection bias is also likely to come into play here, she added, in that "happier people are more likely to marry each other, and less happy people are less likely to get married."

Hopelessness and Resilience

The finding that people who believe "hard work gets one ahead" have higher levels of well-being became an impetus for Graham's later work, which looks at optimism and despair in contemporary America.

Standard economic indicators at the time of the March 2020 *Sharing Knowledge* conference painted a rosy picture, with growth in the stock market and an official unemployment rate of only 3.8 percent.[3] Beginning just a few weeks later, however, the coronavirus pandemic had profoundly altered that picture, threatening economic, health, social, and political systems in the United States and across the world.

While the virus abruptly changed the domestic landscape, many people in the United States had been struggling even before it appeared. Twenty percent of men ages 25 to 54 were not in the labor force largely because they were discouraged or had given up, Graham noted, and so were not counted among the unemployed. There is "an underlying crisis of ill-being and despair that standard economic numbers don't pick up," she asserted.

Other economists reported similar concerns. Princeton University's Anne Case and Angus Deaton have described "deaths of despair" driven by addiction, depression, and suicide among middle-aged White American men without a college degree, findings detailed in a 2015 paper published by the National Academy of Sciences[4] and in the inaugural volume of the *Culture of Health* series.[5] Premature death among that population increased the overall mortality rate in the United States for several consecutive years, even as rates dropped among Black and Latino Americans. (Latino is used here as an inclusive term to include women, men, and non-binary people. The intersectional term *Latinx* is used elsewhere in that volume when it reflects the language of the researchers.)

"We are the only country in the world with a trend this stark in terms of mortality going in the wrong direction," Graham said. While overall life expectancy in the United States did increase in 2018, the small but encouraging shift of 0.1 percent (from 78.6 in 2017 to 78.7 in 2018) does not necessarily indicate a continuing turnaround.[6]

The Pursuit of Happiness

To understand the impact of bifurcated economic and cultural trends in the United States, Graham drew from the body of literature that suggests optimism contributes significantly to longer and happier lives. That raises the question:

"Is the pursuit of happiness equally available to everyone?" She asserted that it is not.

In one longitudinal analysis, Graham used data from the Panel Study of Income Dynamics (PSID) to ascertain levels of optimism among a cohort of people born in the United States in the 1930s and 1940s through 2015.[7] The PSID surveys a nationally representative sample of the same families through much of their lives.

She found that optimistic people live longer, and that optimism better predicts longevity than income, even after controlling for health and other factors. Optimism is also positively associated with socioeconomic status.

Whites with less than a college degree increasingly seem to lack that optimism. Loss of hope in that population appeared as early as the 1970s, Graham noted, a harbinger of the rise in mortality rates today. At the same time, the effects of the civil rights and women's movements of the era were reflected in greater optimism reported by non-Whites and women.

In a separate analysis of responses to the Gallup-Sharecare Global Poll from 2010 to 2015, Graham found that poor Blacks were 2.81 times more likely than poor Whites to say they were optimistic (defined as how they predict their life satisfaction five years into the future), and poor Latinos were 1.21 times more likely than poor Whites to say they were optimistic.[8] The Gallup-Sharecare Global Poll measures people's purpose and social, financial, community, and physical well-being.

Resilience born of cultures that place high value on strong family ties, religious beliefs, and informal support systems may contribute to this heightened optimism, Graham observed, noting that Black and Hispanic respondents report deeper networks of support than Whites.

Hard-won but unfinished progress by Blacks in earnings and longevity may play a role as well: Black males earned 69 percent of the median wages of White males in 1970, a figure that rose to 75 percent by 2013, and the longevity gap between Blacks and Whites narrowed from seven years in 1990 to three in 2014.[9]

Well-Being in Action

Taking a page from the growing interest in models that go beyond standard economic indexes, Santa Monica, located west of downtown Los Angeles, became the first city in the United States to measure the well-being of its residents. But it has done much more than measure: Santa Monica is also incorporating the findings into its framework for government policymaking and performance management.

That work again illustrates that stories and numbers can work hand in hand to build a case for policy change. In this case, anecdotes were the starting point for deciding which data to collect. Several youth-related tragedies between 2009 and 2012 had prompted Santa Monica to ask a question that local governments often fail to consider. Having made significant investments in early childhood, education, youth development, and mental health programs, the city wanted to know: "Is anyone better off as a result?" And it wanted that answer to be based on data, according to Julia E. Rusk, who holds the unique title of Santa Monica's chief of civic well-being.

During focus groups and workshops asking what they valued most, residents talked about wanting their children to thrive, be emotionally and socially capable and resilient, and lead a good life. Those conversations led to the creation of a Youth Wellbeing Report Card, which tracked metrics such as third-grade reading levels and state physical fitness test scores. But it also sparked the recognition that success on individual markers is only part of achieving the overall well-being of Santa Monica's youth and families.

An opportunity to accomplish broader goals came in 2013, when Bloomberg Philanthropies named Santa Monica one of five winners of its Mayors Challenge, an ideas competition that promotes data-driven, high-impact solutions to improve life for city residents. Santa Monica was selected by Bloomberg Philanthropies "for its data-driven approach to measuring and managing well-being in a local context."[10]

Supported by the $1 million prize, the city designed a comprehensive "Local Wellbeing Index," in partnership with RAND Corporation, the New Economics Foundation, a panel of experts, and others.

The goals were to mine research and best practices, findings from periodic resident surveys, and other data sources to develop a multidimensional, people-centered index and local government framework for Santa Monica's budget and its performance management and goals. By combining different types of data, the index would provide insights that could spur policies, programs, and partnerships designed to improve community and individual outcomes.

Findings from the Wellbeing Index, initially released in 2015 and conducted every two years since (most recently in 2019[11]) have six dimensions:

- *Community*: How strong is the sense of community and connection?
- *Place and planet*: Do the built and natural environments support and promote well-being?
- *Learning*: Do people have the opportunity to enrich their knowledge and skill sets across their life span?
- *Health*: How healthy is Santa Monica—physically and mentally?

- *Economic opportunity*: Can a diverse population live and thrive in Santa Monica?
- *Individual outlook*: How do individual residents view their own level of well-being?

What is important is that the community led the city to all this, as opposed to the city leading the community to it.—Julia E. Rusk

Index results indicate that many residents, especially younger ones, increasingly struggle with stress, social isolation, and economic concerns. Latino residents, in particular, are worried about being able to pay for housing, and the number of people who believe the community is becoming unaffordable is growing. At the same time, many seniors are flourishing—yet some are quite vulnerable.

Some of these results have been eye-opening, given Santa Monica's image as an upscale, forward-thinking beach community. Officials believe the insights offered by the Wellbeing Index have helped the city respond to its diverse community, as two local initiatives—the Pico Wellbeing Project and the Wellbeing Microgrants—illustrate.

From Zoning to Economic Opportunity

Direction from the city council to consider zoning needs in Santa Monica's Pico neighborhood provided an opening to apply the city's new way of doing business. Community leaders, many who had led the youth well-being and equity-focused work in Santa Monica, noted the potential impact on gentrification, displacement, and economic opportunity and asked the planning commission and city council to take a fresh approach to the process, drawing on input "from a broader and deeper set of voices," said Rusk. "This well-being work is fundamentally a 'do-different' approach and not solely about measurement. It's about new ways of forging partnerships across sectors, between residents and their government and the many partner organizations."

To develop a shared understanding, community members and city planning staff came together in formats they had not used before. The first step of the Pico Wellbeing Project was to create a community timeline that marks significant neighborhood and community changes illustrating economic, social, political, and cultural realities and future aspirations. That was followed by an "Ideas Sprint"—energetic brainstorming of new solutions to community issues.

Finally, a series of small-scale local conversations, or "coffee chats," enabled small groups of people to provide more informal input.

From its inception, the project has been committed to hearing from everyone who wanted to contribute, so that all had a stake in the outcome. Activities have been conducted in both English and Spanish. Having some sessions conducted in Spanish with non-Spanish speakers wearing headsets for interpretation, was "a very intentional strategy," Rusk noted. "It set a tone from the start that we are serious about broadening the input and making sure we hear from everyone."

This ongoing effort has been neither easy nor quick. Some people have been frustrated by the pace of progress, but others have become involved in city processes in ways they would not previously have believed possible. And the work has gone substantially beyond zoning changes, with the stakeholders creating new economic initiatives to ensure that residents are not displaced.

The project has resulted in the very thing we intended, which is not just to do zoning, but to push the government to be a good actor and partner in focusing resources on new solutions to equitably address community well-being.—Julia E. Rusk

Microgrants to Promote Well-Being

After being named a 2016 winner of the Robert Wood Johnson Foundation (RWJF) Culture of Health prize, Santa Monica used some of the funds to award eight small grants (up to $500 apiece) to community groups to take actions designed to improve community well-being. Twenty-six of these actions had reached 668 people as of December 2019. Examples include:

- A workshop to teach people to make jewelry, get a business license, and sell jewelry in stores
- A clean-up effort in a local park that cleared 1,000 pounds of trash
- The first Black-Creole-owned beauty supply store in Santa Monica
- A financial literacy course for school-age children

Broadening involvement and voices is ultimately what matters—and seeing the impact and power of those voices. So often, people like this, who have really amazing ideas and insights, just get completely overlooked.—Julia E. Rusk

Sharing Stories to Empower
Indigenous Communities

From Central America comes another example of inclusive narrative as a strategic agent of change. While RWJF's work focuses on the United States, in recent years it has looked beyond U.S. borders for lessons that can inform its grantmaking. One set emerges from Guatemala, where Walter Flores and his colleagues at the Center for the Study of Equity and Governance in Health Systems (CEGSS) are raising the profile of Indigenous people and using their stories to strengthen the nation's public health services.

Guatemala has a population of 17.6 million people, a high proportion of whom are Indigenous. Almost three-quarters of that group (73%) live in poverty, compared to 35 percent of non-Indigenous Guatemalans.[12] While all citizens have a government-guaranteed right to health care, the availability of services is often woefully lacking, especially in poor, rural areas.

In a career dedicated to assisting marginalized people in some 30 countries, Flores has seen that governments rarely change policies on the basis of rigorous evidence alone. Reflecting on his early experiences, he explained, "I found myself going back to the same countries over and over to repeat the same message." Looking to do things differently, Flores returned to his native Guatemala to start "a process of more democratic governance of health systems that was very local" and founded CEGSS in 2009 to formalize that work.

To learn more about problems in delivering public health services (e.g., lack of medications, clinics closed due to worker absence, abusive treatment), Flores and his team conducted 25-page, randomized surveys of Indigenous people across the country. But when they presented their written findings, the health authorities paid no attention. Indeed, they suspected that the privileged urban professionals who were collecting data in poor, rural communities were politically motivated.

CEGSS moved to much briefer surveys, with data collected by trained community members, but saw little improvement—few residents had sufficient education to use the surveys and authorities paid only slightly more attention to them.

New Methods, Better Outcomes

Revisiting its strategy, CEGSS began to engage directly with the Indigenous populations. Recognizing that its well-meaning but top-down efforts had perhaps been a bit patronizing, the team took a new tack. Aware that Indigenous communities work through stories and oral communication, they shifted to methods used in anthropology and ethnography, collecting stories from people who had experienced serious hardship because they could not obtain health services.

Echoing the research experience of Carol Graham on well-being, project staff discovered that participants perceived their own circumstances very differently than staff had assumed. The primary complaint of the people they hoped to serve was not lack of access to health services but lack of interest in what matters to them. "We are not treated with respect, with dignity, and there are no efforts to ask *us* [author's emphasis] what we need," they lamented, indicating that their first priority was to have their voices heard.

But gathering the stories consumed time and resources, limiting how many could be collected and making it easier for authorities to discount them as isolated cases. A method was needed to expedite information-gathering.

In rural areas, most families have at least one mobile phone. In 2014, in partnership with community residents, the team launched an SMS message texting platform, which offers a secure way to deliver complaints and readily allows trends to be identified.[13]

The addition of videography and photography made it even easier to tell stories. The team provided community members with voice recorders, smartphones, and cameras to record their testimonies and upload videos to an online platform. The resulting recordings are authentic and compelling, making them more difficult for authorities to ignore. The open access platform has also attracted the attention of journalists—a further inducement for authorities to take action. "We started to see high participation by community members and high response from authorities," Flores reported.

Defending the Right to Health

Through a network established by CEGSS, more than 130 Community Defenders of the Right to Health in 30 Guatemalan municipalities organize and present the information collected by local residents. These community-elected volunteer defenders build on a long-standing principle of solidarity that has enabled Indigenous people to survive centuries of repression. While CEGSS staff provides training and technical assistance, the defenders actually engage with authorities.

The influence of this network has reached beyond the county to state and national levels, where much of the available resources are controlled. The hope is that by working at the national level, structural problems can be more readily fixed in a way that will benefit all rural communities. Despite roadblocks, the defenders have gained access to some very high-level officials and achieved results. CEGSS has produced two short documentaries that showcase the work of the defenders; these documentaries are available on YouTube.[14,15]

Unlike researchers, who can sometimes be brushed off as politicians in disguise, "when somebody living in those territories goes all the way to the capital city to bring their problems, the authorities don't have any other argument. They have to listen to them," said Flores, describing what he has witnessed. Shifting to community-led storytelling has made all the difference in increasing official response and action.[16]

> County and state officers respond when those affected by the problem organize, mobilize, and confront them with evidence. It's not only having rigorous evidence, but who is developing that evidence and whether they feel empowered to engage with authorities.—Walter Flores

Local health services have improved in almost all of the municipalities in which CEGSS works, and governments have allocated more resources to clinics. And, since residents have become more aware of their rights and more willing to report bribery and discrimination, "Bribery has almost disappeared and health care providers are treating them better," said Flores. More communities are actively documenting problems and pushing for improvement, clear that they will not surrender the independence they have developed or allow others to lead or speak for them.

The methods used by CEGSS can be applied, with some modifications, "in any context where there are historically marginalized populations and some rural law or rules and regulations that would allow this to work," stressed Flores. CEGSS is already supporting organizations in India and Peru to replicate its approach.

> Each individual has a story that they want listened to. And they want to spread their own story.—Walter Flores

Shifting Cultural Norms

As with Walter Flores, allowing people to speak for themselves is an important theme to Mallika Dutt, an attorney by training, who advocates for positive change in her home countries of India and the United States, and elsewhere. And like Carol Graham, she is comfortable incorporating human emotions into her work.

Inspired by her involvement with an award-winning music video that educated television viewers in India about domestic violence "by speaking to their emotions and hearts," Dutt left her position in the New Delhi office of the Ford Foundation in 2000 to launch Breakthrough. A global organization, Breakthrough uses arts, media, and technology, along with community mobilization, to inspire people to take action to prevent violence against women and girls.

We have a tendency in the nonprofit world to go on and on about data and outcomes, but that is not the kind of language that moves people. What reaches people is evocative storytelling.—Mallika Dutt

Changing Narratives to Prevent Violence Against Women in India

One of Breakthrough's early campaigns focused on changing public understanding of HIV/AIDS among women in India. While about 80 percent had been infected by their husbands or partners, popular narrative held that most infected women were sex workers.

Working with Positive Women's Network (an Indian network of HIV-positive women) and an advertising agency, Breakthrough created PSA featuring vignettes that showed women's vulnerability to HIV/AIDS in marriage. More than 60 million people watched at least one of the vignettes, which appeared during prime-time family television viewing hours. While the stories resonated with viewers, feedback also pointed to some limitations, Dutt recalled.

After talking with women about the issues, she realized that "shaming men into acting differently was not the best approach." The underlying problem, they told Dutt, was not HIV, but rather "that we have no ability to navigate our personal, sexual, or other safety in our own homes." The partners regrouped and changed their message.

The result was Bell Bajao (Ring the Bell), a multimedia campaign that began with a man overhearing a disturbing episode of domestic violence in an adjacent apartment. Hesitating briefly, he walks to the apartment and rings the doorbell. The noise stops, and the husband angrily opens the door. In a mild voice, the neighbor says only, "Can I get some milk?" When the husband returns with that cup of milk, the neighbor is gone, but the interruption was enough to diffuse the situation. The PSA launched in three languages in 2005 and is available on YouTube (www.youtube.com/watch?v=9t3BPv8tBP4).

Subsequent PSAs (also available on the Breakthrough website), billboards, radio campaigns, and community events introduced other methods of violence interruption, some featuring young boys as disrupters. In the stories, a male character comes upon a threatening situation and diffuses it, giving the viewing public an alternative narrative of what it means to be a man in India.

"Everything changed" when that campaign aired, Dutt said. "The entire country was telling everybody to 'bell bajao.'" In rural areas without doorbells, people substituted, "There's a snake in your house!" The videos went viral, appearing in episodes of four soap operas and as a question on the Indian equivalent of television's *Who Wants to Be a Millionaire?* Regional drama, poetry, and debating competitions used Ring the Bell as a theme to interrupt violence.

Breakthrough's campaign expanded to "Ring the bell. One million men. One million promises,"[17] a global call to men to prevent gender-based violence. As a result, IndiGo Airlines established a no-sexual-harassment policy, and Google's operation in India committed to investing in women-led new tech companies.

"We saw the shift when we moved from a narrative that identified harm to a narrative that invited action and a vision of our desired future," Dutt said. "People were moved by the story and had a clear path to action that they could take to challenge violence against women."

Ingredients for Creating Stories that Resonate

When stories work, Dutt likens them to an orchestra in which multiple voices, sounds, and rhythms come together in harmony. Too often, though, "We practitioners and researchers don't see our own blinders, which prevents us from being in the mystery of creation. We need our right and left brains to come together in a dance for effective storytelling and narrative."

> *There is data and then there is gut, and there is knowing and there is taking a chance.*—Mallika Dutt

Dutt credits a complex mix of data, instinct, creativity, and partnerships for a successful message:

Data: When accurate scientific information informs a storyline, the public has an unbiased framework for understanding a social problem. Other data come from television stations and advertising agencies, which provide feedback about audience size, content recall, and campaign impact. And Breakthrough evaluators survey viewers to learn how well they retain messages and what actions they inspire. With the explosion in mobile technology, community residents have been trained in using their mobile devices to participate in gathering data and tracking progress.

Instinct and creativity: Developing effective stories involves a deep level of listening and honesty and a keen instinct about how far to push a point.

Bell Bajao, for example, pivots on the interaction between two men at a tense moment. Although some women "insisted that the man ringing the bell confront the offender and directly address the violence," Dutt recalled. "All audience research told us that if you asked men to do that, no one would ring the bell."

Partnerships: Dutt often starts a project by asking, "Who in this ecosystem needs to be a lever for change?" and recruits those people as partners and co-creators.

Advertising agencies became important partners, Dutt said, because they "create stories all the time to get us to buy things, and they are brilliant at it." Ad agencies and media outlets came together with Breakthrough staff and constituents in lively and sometimes tense brainstorming sessions. Multiple ideas and storyboards were presented, modified, and rejected before agreement emerged.

Public officials are also key partners. The Bell Bajao campaign was timed to coincide with the introduction of domestic violence legislation in India, for example. Although India has many laws that protect women and girls, they are frequently ignored, Dutt noted. That makes working with government agencies essential to ensure that change happens on the ground and not solely on paper.

Connections with people who are most affected by norms that need to be changed is perhaps the most important partnership. People need to see people who look and act like them in a story. "Peer storytelling is the most powerful way of engaging people on a journey," Dutt said. "More powerful than hearing something from a celebrity."

A Final Word

As the contributors to this chapter show, people can tell their own stories, and academics and others can support those stories with data reflecting their experiences and can help build resilience and foster well-being in any setting— whether a California beach community, a rural village in Guatemala, or a heavily-populated city in India. Each contributor views well-being through a slightly different lens, reflecting the unique concerns of the individuals and communities they serve. But the common thread in this chapter, as throughout the opening part of the book, is that the right blend of story and data—again, the music and the math—can foster the narrative change that propels a Culture of Health forward.

A New Narrative on Gun Violence

Bernadette Callahan Hohl, PhD, MPH, Assistant Professor, Department of Biostatistics and Epidemiology; Co-Director, New Jersey Center on Gun Violence Research at Rutgers University, Rutgers University School of Public Health

Michael B. Siegel, MD, MPH, Professor, Department of Community Health Sciences, Boston University School of Public Health

Daniel W. Webster, ScD, MPH, Bloomberg Professor of American Health; Director, Johns Hopkins Center for Gun Policy and Research, Bloomberg School of Public Health, Johns Hopkins University

Gun violence, made visible by the near-constant, almost daily news reports of shootings, is perhaps as ripe for narrative change as any social or health issue of our time. At this divisive moment in our nation's history, the tragedy of gun injuries and deaths seems only to inflame the rhetoric that separates Americans, rather than lead to a shared policy agenda.

The discordance is often traced to the Second Amendment to the Constitution, which reads, "A well-regulated Militia, being necessary to the security of a free State, the right of the people to keep and bear Arms, shall not be infringed." This sentence has been a touchstone that has too often precluded civil conversation and productive debate. Conflicting interpretations of its intent and polarizing statements from industry and other narrow-interest groups have created a false narrative that obscures sound evidence supporting widely shared gun violence policies.

> *It is a myth that gun violence prevention and the Second Amendment are mutually exclusive. That is not the case.*—Michael B. Siegel

The contributors to this chapter offer an alternative narrative drawing from public health tenets and practice. Here, public discourse follows from evidence

Bernadette Callahan Hohl, Michael B. Siegel, and Daniel W. Webster, *A New Narrative on Gun Violence* In: *Community Resilience*. Edited by: Alonzo L. Plough, Oxford University Press (2021). © Robert Wood Johnson Foundation.
DOI: 10.1093/oso/9780197559383.003.0004

indicating that there is no monolithic "gun culture," and that gun control and gun rights advocates agree in some significant areas.

Importantly, the contributors demonstrate that the most effective policies for reducing gun violence are not only the least invasive but also those where gun owners and non-owners tend to agree. Their work offers a road map that allows room for philosophical differences while offering guidance on how people can act together in their shared interest of preventing tragic deaths.

Boston University's Michael B. Siegel turned his attention to gun policy in the aftermath of the 2012 shootings in the small town of Sandy Hook, Conn., near his childhood home of Danbury. He engages his co-contributors in a discussion of public health principles that can shape thinking about guns and gun policy and describes studies that apply those principles.

Drawing from his experiences in Baltimore, Daniel W. Webster of Johns Hopkins University illustrates how gun violence has influenced urban life, examining the implications of aggressive law enforcement and the use of harsh criminal penalties. His work with police and community members in Baltimore and his involvement with a gun violence reduction consortium yield practical strategies for reducing harm.

Zeroing in on the community environments in which gun violence occurs, Bernadette Callahan Hohl at the New Jersey Center on Gun Violence Research illustrates how a public health approach can improve safety and well-being. Using examples from community-driven projects, including efforts to "green" abandoned lots, she offers evidence that strengthening neighborhoods pays off.

Following a short summary of data on gun ownership, gun-related deaths, and public opinions about gun policy, this chapter presents a conversation among the contributors about principles that can enrich the narrative and inform policies. The chapter concludes with examples from each contributor's work that demonstrate how those principles can be applied and suggests an action agenda.

Gun Ownership, Fatalities, and Public Opinion

Data about gun ownership and gun violence are inadequate and at times confusing and unreliable. Federal legislation dating to 1996 effectively precluded the nonpartisan Centers for Disease Control and Prevention (CDC) from addressing gun control, and the agency has not measured gun ownership since 2004.

To compensate, researchers have turned to survey responses and proxy measures to estimate gun ownership, while police records, death certificates, and FBI reports have provided information about gun fatalities. Together these sources yield a general, if incomplete, picture of guns in the United States. Here is some of what we know.

Gun Ownership

Most people who exercise their right to own a gun do so legally and responsibly. Gun ownership for many is an important part of their lives: Nearly three-quarters of gun owners reported they could never see themselves *not* owning a gun, according to a report from the Pew Research Center.[1]

Three out of every 10 Americans own at least one firearm, according to the Pew report, and two-thirds of gun owners have more than one. With 393.3 million guns in circulation, there are 90 million more guns than people in the United States.[2]

The National Rifle Association (NRA), a gun rights advocacy organization, was established in 1871 to "promote and encourage rifle shooting on a scientific basis," according to Col. William C. Church, one of its founders.[3] It also has a tradition of providing firearm education programs.

With its significant presence in gun policy debates, the NRA has been viewed as the voice of gun owners in the United States, although only 19 percent of them reported being NRA members in 2017. While it has been in some turmoil in recent years, marked by the ouster of its president and litigation over its tax-exempt status, the NRA remains a powerful policy and advocacy force.

Gun-Related Homicides

Guns are a significant cause of fatalities in the United States. Nearly 40,000 residents died from gun violence in 2017, the most since at least 1968, the earliest year for which the CDC has online data.[4] Homicides and suicides accounted for 16.4 percent of all fatal injuries that year.[5] Blacks are eight times more likely than Whites to be firearm-related homicide victims.[6,7]

Causes of Gun Fatalities in the United States: 2018

Suicides	24,432
Homicides	13,958
Law enforcement involved	539
Unintentional	438
Undetermined	353
Total Fatalities	39,720

When the type of firearm is specified in police reports for homicides, nearly 92 percent were handguns, 4 percent were rifles, 3 percent were shotguns, and 2 percent were "other."[8] The FBI statistics do not capture all gun homicides, however, because they rely on reports from state and local police departments, some of which do not participate or provide only incomplete information.

Opinions on Gun Policy

The evidence of common ground across ideological lines and gun ownership status suggests opportunities for deeper discussion and policy development while the areas of disagreement highlight a need for unbiased research.[9]

Public Opinion on Select Gun Policies

Policy Issues of Significant or Moderate Agreement

In favor of background checks for private sales and sales at gun shows	77% of gun owners 87% of non-gun owners
In favor of barring people on no-fly or watch lists from purchasing guns	82% of gun owners 84% of non-gun owners
In favor of allowing people to carry a concealed firearm without a permit	33% of gun owners 12% of non-gun owners
In favor of barring people with mental illness from purchasing guns	89% of gun owners 89% of non-gun owners

Policy Issues of Disagreement

In favor of a federal database to track gun sales	54% of gun owners 80% of non-gun owners
In favor of banning assault weapons	48% of gun owners 77% of non-gun owners
Belief that gun violence is a major problem in the country today	33% of gun owners 59% of non-gun owners

The Pew Research Center reports significant differences in opinions according to party affiliation. Republican gun owners, for example, were about twice as likely as Democratic gun owners to say that owning a gun is essential to their freedom (91% compared with 43%). But areas of agreement across party lines are also striking:

- Most (93%) Democrats and Republicans (82%) reported being in favor of background checks for private gun sales and sales at gun shows.[10]

- Nearly 90 percent (89%) of Democrats and nearly 80 percent (78%) of Republicans favor barring gun purchases from people on no-fly or watch lists.[11]
- More than 90 percent (91%) of respondents from both parties favor preventing people with mental illness from buying guns.[12]

The opinions related to gun ownership among people with mental illness, widely shared among gun owners, non-owners, Republicans, and Democrats, suggest an area for further research, as evidence suggests that mental illness is a weak predictor of violent behavior. This issue is addressed in a further section of this chapter, under the heading "Assessing and Reducing Risk Factors for Violence."

A Public Health Perspective on Gun Violence

The public health field has the expertise to provide evidence that will enrich the knowledge base on gun policy. To frame that expertise, Michael B. Siegel introduced four core public health tenets that offer insights into the causes and effects of gun violence; observations from other chapter contributors are also incorporated into this section.

Siegel's four tenets are built around the social ecological model; the epidemiologic triad; population health and health disparities; and the well-being of the public.

A Social Ecological Model

The public health social ecological model[13] situates individuals in a circle surrounded by ever-larger circles of the social, built, and natural environments. Gun violence problems have often been defined at the level of the innermost circle—a specific violent perpetrator or a "few bad apples in the police department," as Siegel describes it. Gun violence problems framed this way yield responses focused on individuals, such as incarcerating perpetrators or better training for police officers. Because they overlook context, these responses fail to address underlying sources of the problem.

Daniel W. Webster commented on the limits of that narrow perspective by recalling Baltimore in the predigital era. "You would walk into the police department and see red pins on a map indicating where shootings took place. The good news was that you could see the environmental risk. The bad news was that the response was to send a lot of police into the areas where the dots were most connected. Even in neighborhoods where there were a lot of red pins on the map, however, the vast majority of residents are not dangerous."

Policies such as broad stop and frisk; aggressive racially-based arrests, prosecution, and sentencing for drug possession; and subjecting juveniles to harsh adult criminal justice systems create lasting harms and have been used as tools of oppression.—Daniel W. Webster

Aggressive law enforcement responses to neighborhood incidents may actually cause gun violence rather than reduce it, Webster observes, because public trust is critical to public safety. The April 2015 death of Freddie Gray while in police custody in Baltimore did not involve a firearm, but after the subsequent civil unrest, "The rates of homicides and shootings almost doubled," he said. According to a tally compiled by the *Baltimore Sun*, shooting deaths in Baltimore rose from 160 in 2014 to 299 in 2015. With 309 shooting deaths in 2019, that trend appears to have flattened but not decreased.[14]

Reflecting on her community-based violence prevention work, Bernadette Callahan Hohl suggests that public health professionals could be more effective if they put gun violence in a larger context of social determinants (the economic and social conditions in the places where people live, learn, work, and play), rather than accepting the traditional focus on individual culprits. The struggle, she says, reflects in part the way the problem has been defined.

Findings from Siegel's study of fatal police shootings[15] amplify Hohl's call for attention to context. The Black-White racial disparity here is widely recognized, but the magnitude of the disparity varies greatly across cities. To understand why, Siegel analyzed those shootings in 69 large U.S. cities from 2013 to 2017. The ratios ranged from a low of 0.0 (no disparity) to a high of 46.7, a difference that could not be attributed to racial bias by individual police officers alone, he says.

After controlling for each city's crime rates, Black median income, size, racial composition of its police force, and other factors, Siegel found that the level of residential segregation was significantly associated with the magnitude of the racial disparity in fatal police shootings.

What police need to be trained in is not merely how to treat individuals differently, but to recognize that they police Black neighborhoods differently.—Michael B. Siegel

The Epidemiologic Triad

Public health uses the epidemiologic triad model to examine the interactions between a "host" (the patient, or here the victim of gun violence); an agent (the microorganism that causes the disease, or here the gun); and a vector (the organism that transmits the disease, or here the gun manufacturer and gun lobby).

Responses to gun violence have focused largely on the host, Siegel realized, so he began to explore the agent and the vector. Analyzing trends in gun manufacturing and gun legislation, he found a spike in the production of firearms in 2005, fueled mainly by an increase in lethal, higher caliber pistols and in rifles. That same year, Florida passed the nation's first "stand-your-ground" law, which allows the use of lethal force even where it might have been possible to retreat safely. Both gun production and stand-your-ground laws were "driven by a direct effort by the NRA to convince people they were in danger," he says.

Improving Population Health and Reducing Health Disparities

One particularly troubling aspect of the current skewed gun narrative is its failure to recognize the disproportionate effect that gun violence has on communities where residents already suffer from a host of structural inequities. "Mass shootings get publicized, but what is killing the most people are the everyday shootings that take place largely in an urban environment and that largely affect communities of color, especially Black communities," explains Siegel.

The third tenet in Siegel's framework is that gun violence is a structural problem that affects some populations more than others. As such, this tenet guides stakeholders to policies that consider underlying disparities, such as poverty and the kind of neighborhood-level segregation that drives differences in police-involved fatalities.

Promoting the Well-Being of the Public

The fourth public health tenet holds that the client is the public, including gun rights and gun control advocates alike.

The debate has been framed as gun owners vs. non-gun owners, but the public is comprised of both, and gun owners and non-gun owners do not need to be pitted against each other.—Michael B. Siegel

The public health field in general knows little about gun owners, Siegel acknowledges: "We have traditionally kind of left them aside and focused on what we can do to protect non-gun owners." This posture inevitably alienates responsible gun owners and makes them feel scapegoated by people they believe know nothing about guns yet are trying to regulate their behavior. "That is neither effective nor inclusive," he says.

It is also at odds with the mission and tactics of public health. Through its systematic approach, the field is charged with seeking unbiased answers that do not favor one portion of the population over another. An emphasis on the harm caused by guns, rather than the guns themselves, brings that perspective to the fore.

"When you attend public hearings," Siegel notes, "non-gun owners get up and speak about background checks or keeping guns out of the wrong hands. Then, gun owners get up and speak about Second Amendment rights. Why don't you see them speaking together, when most gun owners support the policies the non-owners had just advocated?"

Bringing gun owners and non-owners together in common cause would be a game-changing accomplishment.—Michael B. Siegel

Building a Culture of Health Around Firearm Violence

Within the discipline they share, Siegel, Webster, and Hohl pursue their own research into gun violence reduction; highlights of each person's work are summarized in this section.

Michael B. Siegel: Two Studies Suggest a Path Forward

With support from the Robert Wood Johnson Foundation (RWJF), Siegel and co-investigator Claire Boine, a research scholar at the Boston University School of Public Health, are conducting two studies aimed at informing a Culture of Health as it relates to firearm violence.

A Study of Gun Culture and State Gun Laws

Their first study, conducted in two parts, unpacked the so-called gun culture and examined the relative effectiveness of select gun policies. Findings have appeared in the *Annals of Internal Medicine*,[16] *American Journal of Public Health*,[17] and the *Journal of General Internal Medicine*.[18] "We tend to think of culture as something that just kind of happens naturally," Siegel says, but powerful private interests can have a very intentional influence on narratives about culture.

Siegel and Boine analyzed 10 state-level variables hypothesized to reflect different gun subcultures: the proportions of NRA members and of hunters in the state; per capita numbers of federally licensed gun dealers and of military enlistments; the presence of a stand-your-ground law; per capita numbers of handgun and of long gun background checks; per capita subscriptions to *Guns and Ammo* magazine; the proportion of NRA members who subscribe to the *American Hunter* magazine; and the proportion of members who subscribe to *America's 1st Freedom*, the magazine of the NRA.

> *Gun owners do not comprise a single culture.*—Michael B. Siegel

Siegel and Boine's research placed owners into three discrete subcultures: a subculture of hunting and target shooting, a subculture of self-defense, and a subculture holding that guns are an important symbol of freedom. They found that only the third group—the subculture of freedom—was associated with higher rates of homicide. They also found that the greater presence of a hunting subculture was associated with lower rates of firearm homicide.

> *The major elements of gun culture such as hunting, collecting, target shooting, and self-defense are compatible with building a Culture of Health around firearms.*—Michael B. Siegel

The agenda, then, should not be framed as a battle between gun owners and non-owners but rather as collective action to unite around shared values. "This is the least controversial area I have ever worked in," Siegel declares. That assertion might be startling, but Siegel notes that he had found more support for universal background checks for gun ownership than he had for cigarette taxes or smoke-free restaurants when he was studying tobacco policies in the 1990s and early 2000s. Indeed, to emphasize his point, he notes that "more people support universal background checks than believe the earth revolves around the sun."

To analyze the effectiveness of select gun policies, Siegel and Boine linked information from a state database of gun laws (www.statefirearmlaws.org) to state data on firearm violence and sociodemographic variables from 1991 to 2016. They found that laws regulating the *types* of firearms that are permissible are not associated with lower homicide rates at the state level, but laws regulating *who* may possess a weapon are, and significantly so:

- Universal background checks are associated with a 16.1 percent reduction in overall firearm homicide rates.
- Laws requiring people subject to domestic violence restraining orders to relinquish their firearms are associated with a 14 percent drop in firearm-related intimate partner homicide rates.
- Restricting gun possession by people with a history of conviction for a violent misdemeanor is associated with a 20 percent reduction in homicide rates.
- Laws that ban assault weapons are not associated with lower homicide rates.

- "Shall issue" laws, which prohibit police discretion in granting concealed carry permits, are associated with an 8.6 percent increase in homicide rates.

A Common Agenda for Gun Owners and Non-Owners

In the second study, which runs until December 2021, Siegel and Boine are digging more deeply into the attitudes, beliefs, and practices of gun owners. This study includes a survey and focus groups with a broad spectrum of gun owners: hunters and people who visit shooting ranges, people who own guns for self-defense, people who believe they have to protect themselves from the government, and individuals who have contemplated suicide. "We are for the first time acknowledging that there are different types of gun owners, that gun culture is not monolithic," Siegel says in describing the study.

Their ultimate goal is to bring gun owners and non-owners together in person to develop shared policy agendas that they can jointly present to policymakers, not as "a gun owner community" or a "non-gun owner community" but as collaborators committed to reducing violence without abridging rights.

Hohl looks forward to that effort, acknowledging that people on both sides of the debate have preconceived ideas about one another. "We don't necessarily know who is and isn't a gun owner, and maybe we shouldn't make assumptions."

Daniel W. Webster: Structural Determinants, Risk, and Public Policy

Growing up in rural Kentucky, where his father served as a small-town mayor, Daniel W. Webster was exposed to social problems early in life. And he saw them again, as a young child protective services caseworker, when he was threatened by a gun during an investigation of child abuse in the home.

When Webster moved to Baltimore in the mid-1980s, his exposure to social problems and the risk of guns intensified, as the city was "experiencing an unprecedented and extraordinary rise in homicides involving firearms in young Black males," he recalls. Most of the homicides were associated with substance use, and the principal response was heavy policing and gun and drug laws that led to long periods of incarceration.

The Johns Hopkins Center for Gun Policy and Research

Webster brought those experiences to bear on his work with the Johns Hopkins Center for Gun Policy and Research, which was established in 1995 partly to fill the gap caused by congressional restrictions on gun research in the federal government. The center's multidisciplinary faculty studies the effects of gun laws, generates support for evidence-based gun policies, analyzes law enforcement responses to violence, and advises and evaluates community prevention efforts.

One center study draws from arrest records and community surveys to identify and remove structural barriers to productive relationships between police officers and residents. Although community residents agreed that gun violence is a significant problem and that too many people carry guns, they aren't happy with the law enforcement approach in their communities. "The police arrest everybody but the people who are really the most dangerous," one told Webster.

Police records seem to support that assertion, finding that about half the arrests for illegal gun possession in Baltimore are dismissed without explanation, possibly because many resulted from inappropriate or illegal searches. Residents said they wanted the police to develop more transparent policies within the department and to be clear about who gets stopped on the street, and why. Such actions, they believed, can contribute to better police-community relationships.

> When communities do not trust the police, there is a lot more violence. They don't turn to the police for help; they try to solve the problems themselves through street justice; retaliatory violence.—Daniel W. Webster

Assessing and Reducing Risk Factors for Violence

Webster's work has convinced him that a sophisticated understanding of the underlying structures and social networks that surround people most at risk is essential to creating policies and programs that address those risks.

Institutional racism is one such structure, he maintains, noting that race affects the opportunities people have and the context in which they live. "I think the usual conversation is too narrow," he says. "Race typically comes up in the context of law enforcement, but the underlying problem is the barriers to having a full life." Addressing structural racism, therefore, means that public health has to "get entrenched in what the police are doing."

One mechanism for examining risk is the Consortium for Risk-Based Firearm Policy,[19] of which Webster is a member. An initiative of the nonprofit Educational Fund to Stop Gun Violence, the consortium develops recommendations and creates resources and toolkits for policymakers and practitioners. For example:

- A state legislative toolkit helps states develop extreme risk protection orders.[20] These court-ordered warrants enable family members (often the first to recognize risk) and law enforcement to work together to permanently or temporarily deny access to guns for people at high risk of endangering themselves or others. Research has shown that for every 10 to 20 risk warrants issued, one life is saved.[21] As of July 2019, the District of Columbia and 17 states had enacted some form of risk protection legislation.[22]

- A report, "Guns, Public Health, and Mental Illness,"[23] summarizes the body of evidence demonstrating that despite widely held perceptions, mental illness alone is rarely the cause of violence. Findings from the report might be used to improve public understanding and narrative about mental illness and to suggest targeted areas of intervention. For example, evidence indicates that only four percent of violence in the United States is attributable to mental illness. Domestic violence does increase the risk of firearm violence, however, and mental illnesses, such as depression, significantly increase the risk of suicide.

Webster points to Oakland, California, as one example of an intensive public health intervention strategy designed to go beyond "putting Band-Aids on a gushing wound." Oakland Ceasefire[24] is a structured partnership between community members, social services, and law enforcement dedicated to reducing gun violence and identifying ingredients essential to successful violence reduction. Homicides in Oakland dropped from 126 in 2012, when Oakland Ceasefire began, to 68 in 2018. Nonfatal shootings dropped from 561 to 277 in the same period.

Bernadette Hohl: The Environments in Which People Live

Bernadette Callahan Hohl also uses a public health framework to advance her commitment to reducing violence. As co-director of the New Jersey Center on Gun Violence Research at Rutgers University, she focuses on the impact of regular exposure to gun violence.

Established in 2018, the center provides the state with multidisciplinary research, evidence-based policy recommendations, and strategies for translating evidence into actionable community programs. It is one of only two state-funded gun centers in the country. The state sponsorship provides practical advantages in the form of access to data and program information, and perhaps even more significantly, it has symbolic importance in demonstrating a public commitment to reducing gun violence.

Clean Communities and Safe Open Spaces

Referencing the close ties between gun violence and other social determinants of health, Hohl describes a "complex web of causation" in which poor outcomes in one domain interact with poor outcomes in others. The opposite—the inter-action of positive outcomes—is also important, and Hohl believes that tackling the constellation of challenges that communities identify as priorities "will in turn have an effect on reducing gun violence."

That view is reflected in the comments of residents asked to describe what successful violence prevention means to them. Instead of mentioning guns as their first priority, they often speak of "clean communities, civil neighbors, the ability to engage with their children's schools, and of feeling safe when walking to and from work," Hohl notes.

As researchers seek to disentangle the web of factors that make struggling communities unsafe, they are well advised to build on activities already un-derway, adds Hohl, commenting, "I don't create programs, I find them." She listens to residents' perspectives as to which community-based social, housing, or other programs best address neighborhood needs, takes a systematic approach to assessing their effectiveness, and then feeds that knowledge back to the com-munity. "My drive has always been 'evidence-based practice and practice-based evidence,'" she says.

Researchers are obligated to provide the tools to help people understand whether what they are doing is working, and to alert them to unintended consequences.—Bernadette Callahan Hohl

Greening the Neighborhood

To many people, an overabundance of vacant or abandoned lots may not seem closely related to the problem of gun violence. But they are a critical concern for residents in low-resourced communities and an example of how a seemingly un-related initiative can become a safety guardrail.

Hohl has been collaborating with a team of researchers across the country in evaluating local efforts to convert empty lots into safe and attractive public spaces, providing community residents with qualitative and quantitative evi-dence about their impact. Philadelphia, with more than 40,000 vacant spaces in 2019, is among the communities under study.

There, a community-led "clean-and-green" effort to stabilize and im-prove vacant lots in one neighborhood expanded over time to include sev-eral models of intervention. In one, local landscapers under contract to the Pennsylvania Horticultural Society removed trash, graded the land, added plants, and installed low fences. Evaluators found that "vacant lot greening was associated with reductions in gun assaults, vandalism to surrounding buildings, and stress, and with increases in self-reported levels of physical ac-tivity," says Hohl.

Another evaluation examined compliance with a 2010 ordinance requiring owners of abandoned buildings in Philadelphia to install working doors and windows and to clean the facades. Near to buildings where owners complied with the ordinance, the team found a 39 percent reduction in gun assaults, a 19 percent reduction in other assaults, and a 16 percent reduction in nuisance crimes.

Similar findings emerged from a randomized trial comparing vacant lots that had been greened with lots that lacked greening. Residents living near remediated lots reported reduced perceptions of crime, vandalism, and safety concerns and more use of outside spaces for relaxing and socializing. There were also changes in police-reported outcomes, including significantly less crime. Subsequent analyses demonstrated especially strong outcomes in reducing gun violence.

The research team has also evaluated greening initiatives in Flint, Michigan; New Orleans; and Youngstown, Ohio. From these studies of four distinct communities, which are profiled in an October 2019 article in *Health Affairs*,[25] a broad base of evidence emerges to guide future investments.

Changing Narratives and Outcomes

Reflecting on their research experiences, Hohl, Siegel, and Webster proposed action items to promote greater understanding, thoughtful dialogue, and better outcomes. Across all strategies is a recognition that expanding the narrative to one that engages both gun control and gun rights advocates across the political spectrum and from many disciplines is essential.

Build and Disseminate Data and Findings

The three contributors agreed that issues related to gun ownership and gun violence cry out for more data, better data, data repositories, and data-sharing capacity. Not enough is known about who owns guns and for what purpose, or about the individual and institutional factors that cause people to harm themselves or others. Without that kind of information, it is easy to draw false conclusions based on sensational or unrepresentative stories and to misunderstand or demonize people who hold different views. When that happens, an opportunity to develop a shared narrative that advances evidence-based solutions to the violence that concerns everyone is lost.

A key first step, says Webster, is for researchers and practitioners to share data they already have, both informally and by developing a master inventory of sources. A central database would facilitate research and provide answers to policymakers, many of whom express serious interest in good data. During the primary season, "Staff of five of the 2020 candidates for president asked me for data," Webster says.

Data repositories and inventories should not be limited to numbers and lists, adds Hohl. They should also be able to provide baseline comparisons across groups and to identify population-level patterns and trends.

All cited the "centers of excellence" established and funded by the CDC, which provide resources, training, and guidance on pressing public health issues, as a model. A comparable gun violence center of excellence based at the CDC or elsewhere could serve as a focal point for data, research, and training resources. Siegel calls for a "research base that doesn't say 'does this law work?'" but rather one that asks, "What is the set of laws that will have the greatest impact?"

Diffusion of innovation across states and localities is also important to spread effective public and social policies, emphasizes Siegel. While laws such as extreme risk protection orders and domestic violence restrictions are starting to diffuse, he notes, stand-your-ground laws have actually been the most widely diffused thus far, not necessarily the initiative many would favor.

Explore Pressing Topics

The contributors suggested some specific policy questions that call for further investigation. Better understanding of these issues might promote broader consensus on some sensitive gun policy topics and lead to a more effective public narrative about gun violence.

- What are the implications of a national gun registry? Gun owners fear a registry is the first step to large-scale gun confiscation, while gun-rights advocates believe it is an important management tool. There is no evidence to support or dispute either perspective.
- What strategies are effective in reducing illegal gun possession? Convictions for illegal possession are important drivers of incarceration, says Webster, but there is no solid research on factors such as mandatory minimum sentences for illegal possession and no good models or research on alternatives to incarceration or postincarceration services for people convicted of illegal gun possession.
- What are the consequences of concealed carry laws? Should there be a higher bar for permitting people to carry guns in public than for keeping them in their homes?

- What community-based intensive interventions are working, and how do we support them? Disseminating promising practices with toolkits, technical assistance, and other resources is essential to achieving systemic changes.

A Final Word

The responses to horrific mass shootings, police-involved homicides in Black communities, and gun-related suicides have only laid bare the country's deep divide over guns. Progress seems elusive but as the contributors to this chapter point out, much of the divisive gun violence narrative has been driven by narrow interests and false assumptions rather than on sound research. Their work offers evidence that another narrative, based on solid data and a rigorous research agenda, not only is possible but also has the potential to inform policy proposals that cross personal and political divides.

Major public health victories in vaccine-preventable diseases, motor vehicle safety, tobacco control, and more tell us that we can craft new narratives about prevention and treatment that lead to societal change. The contributors in this chapter throw their disciplinary "hats in the ring" to suggest that public health's involvement in the field of gun violence can also drive a consensus narrative, setting the stage for more effective policies in this arena as well.

Immigrants in America

Stories of Trauma and Resilience

Heather Koball, PhD, Co-Director, National Center for Children in Poverty

Airín D. Martínez, PhD, Assistant Professor, Health Policy & Management, School of Public Health & Health Sciences, University of Massachusetts–Amherst

Francesca Menes, MPA, Founder and Chief Engager, CommUnity Strategies, LLC; Co-Founder and Board Chair, The Black Collective, Inc.

Kate Vickery, MPA, MSCRP, Executive Director, Houston Immigration Legal Services Collaborative

What makes someone "American"? Some identify as American because of the circumstances of their birth. But one out of every seven people living in the United States was not born a U.S. citizen, so many become, or consider themselves, American by other means. As of 2018, there were 44.8 million immigrants who made their home here, and almost three-quarters (73%) have been here for more than 10 years.[1] Most (77%) are in the country as naturalized citizens and lawful permanent residents or hold temporary visas. Another 23 percent lack authorization to remain and are undocumented.[2] Immigrants comprised 17.4 percent of the U.S. labor force in 2018 according to the Bureau of Labor Statistics.[3]

South and East Asian immigrants comprise the largest proportion of the immigrant population (27.4%), followed by Mexicans (25.3%), and other Latin Americans (25.1%). Starting in 2010 and each year since then, more Asian than Latino immigrants have entered the country.[4]

Through research studies and community interventions, the contributors to this chapter illustrate the myriad ways that the immigrant experience is a key

Heather Koball, Airín D. Martínez, Francesca Menes, and Kate Vickery, *Immigrants in America* In: *Community Resilience*. Edited by: Alonzo L. Plough, Oxford University Press (2021). © Robert Wood Johnson Foundation. DOI: 10.1093/oso/9780197559383.003.0005 dimension of American life. Heather Koball of the National Center for Children in Poverty uses national data to better understand how state and federal policies shape the lives of immigrant children and families. She describes two studies that analyze the impacts of immigrant-focused and enforcement-focused policies on the health and material well-being of low-income immigrant families.

In her look at Mexican-origin families in Phoenix, University of Massachusetts–Amherst faculty member Airín D. Martínez examines the effects of racism and antagonistic immigration enforcement policies on family health and stress. Her research method integrates qualitative interviews that garner family self-reports of health with saliva samples that provide biomarkers for chronic disease.

Kate Vickery, who is with the Houston Immigration Legal Services Collaborative, illustrates the importance of collaborative strategies to promote a vibrant immigrant community. Challenged by a high-enforcement environment and battered by Hurricane Harvey, Houston's immigrants nonetheless contribute significantly to the region's culture and economy.

The chapter ends with CommUnity's Francesca Menes's perspectives on Black immigrants, a diverse and understudied population. Menes illustrates how exclusionary public policies and institutional racism criminalize Black immigrants, drawing from her work in Miami to suggest an agenda for action and research.

Immigrant Status Terms

Asylee: A person who meets the definition of refugee, is in the United States or a port of entry and has been granted the rights of asylum status. Asylees are eligible to apply for permanent residence after one year.

Asylum: A legal status sought by noncitizens in the United States who cannot return to their home country due to past persecution or a well-founded fear of future persecution.

DACA recipient: A person covered by Deferred Action for Childhood Arrivals (DACA), a program of temporary deportation relief that provides a two-year work permit and other rights to qualifying young adults who were brought to the United States illegally as children. DACA does not provide a route to citizenship.

Immigrant: A U.S. resident who was born outside the United States to non-American parents, regardless of legal status.

Lawfully permanent resident ("green card" holder): A noncitizen allowed to live permanently in the United States and to work, own property, receive financial tuition assistance, and join the U.S. Armed Forces. Permanent status can be forfeited in certain circumstances.

Refugee: A person living outside his or her home country who cannot return due to past persecution or a well-founded fear of future persecution.

Temporary Protected Status (TPS): Legal permission to remain in the United States temporarily. This status, for nationals of countries designated by the attorney general, is granted for a designated period and can be renewed.

Unauthorized (undocumented) immigrant: A person who is not a U.S. citizen and does not have lawful temporary or permanent status. Unauthorized immigrants may have entered legally (e.g., with a tourist or work visa), but overstayed the terms of the visa (e.g., a student who quits school or a tourist who overstays) or may have entered unlawfully. The terms unauthorized and undocumented are used interchangeably in this chapter.

Immigration Enforcement Policies

E-Verify: An online system in which employers can check the immigration status of their employees, available in all states and mandatory for federal employers and contractors. As of August 2018, more than 750,000 employers were enrolled in E-Verify.[5]

Secure Communities: A program requiring local law enforcement agencies to send fingerprints of anyone they arrest to Department of Homeland Security (DHS) databases. If an immigration violation is found, Immigration, Customs, and Enforcement (ICE) officials may ask local law enforcement to detain the person so that ICE can take custody. Submitting fingerprints is required by law; detaining people pending ICE arrival is not.

287(g): A provision of the 1996 Immigration and Nationality Act that allows jurisdictions to sign memoranda of understanding with ICE, deputizing local law enforcement officials to carry out federal enforcement functions such as investigating, apprehending, and detaining noncitizens. In July 2019, there were 89 jurisdictions in 21 states that participated in a full or limited 287(g) program.[6]

Child Health and Immigration Enforcement

Heather Koball's research on low-income families with young children takes its inspiration from two passions that are not always connected—her principles of faith, which undergird a commitment to caring for the underserved, and her love of math. Her goal, she says, is to use "facts and evidence to shape for the better government policies that disproportionately affect low-income families and children."

About 18 million children in the United States live with at least one parent who was not born here, including 5.3 million who live with an undocumented immigrant. Most (4.5 million) of these children are U.S.-born citizens, while the remainder are themselves undocumented.[7]

Beginning in the late 1990s and early 2000s, states diverged in the extent to which they used their own resources to participate in federal immigration enforcement efforts and to extend social safety net benefits to immigrants without papers. The divergent paths created a natural experiment within which to assess the impact on health. Two studies—one of immigrant-focused policies and one of enforcement-focused policies—examine the effects on children and families.

The Impact of Policies Focused on Immigrants

Koball's study funded by the Robert Wood Johnson Foundation (RWJF) examines whether policies that offer sanctuary to immigrants and that issue driver's licenses to undocumented immigrants increase the chances that children in immigrant families will receive adequate medical and dental care.

The sanctuary policies adopted in some regions limit cooperation with ICE requests to detain undocumented immigrants and the extent to which local police departments participate in federal immigration enforcement. Proponents argue that sanctuary policies promote well-being in that they safeguard Fourth Amendment rights (the constitutional provision against unreasonable search and seizure), maintain trust between law enforcement and immigrant communities, and allocate scarce local law enforcement resources more efficiently.

Access to driver's licenses is another policy that arguably improves safety and helps overcome the transportation barriers that limit access to school, jobs, and health care, all important factors in promoting resilience among families and children. Until 1993, undocumented immigrants could legally obtain a license in every state, but by 2011 all but three states no longer issued them. More recently, some states again began to offer driver's licenses to immigrants. As of December 2019, there were 15 states, the District of Columbia, and Puerto Rico that allowed undocumented immigrants to apply for licenses.[8]

Methods and Findings

To measure the impact of sanctuary and driver's license policies, Koball merged data on state-level immigration policies from 2000 to 2016[9] with data for the same years from the Medical Expenditure Panel Survey (MEPS), a nationally representative survey of the Agency for Healthcare Research and Quality.

The key finding was that children of immigrant parents living in regions that offered sanctuary and driver's licenses were more likely to have a usual source of health care and were significantly less likely to have unmet medical needs than children of immigrants living in regions without these policies.

Sanctuary policies and driver's licenses for undocumented immigrants improved preventive health outcomes among children of immigrants.
—Heather Koball

As one of the next steps in her research, Koball plans to ascertain the immigration status of families living in places with sanctuary and driver's licenses policies and to analyze the effects of those policies on family members according to their legal status.

Aggressive Enforcement and Material Hardship

Koball's second study, funded by the Russell Sage Foundation, tried to anticipate what would happen to both legal and undocumented immigrants in localities that participated aggressively in federal immigration enforcement efforts initiated by the Trump administration. Whatever the consequences, enforcement is clearly having an effect: The number of federal criminal arrests for immigration violations increased by 87 percent in the first full fiscal year of the administration, and criminal prosecutions rose by 66 percent during that period.[10]

This reflected, at least in part, a federal policy change in 2017 that restored the far-reaching Secure Communities program. That initiative had been in effect from 2008 until it was rescinded by President Barack Obama in 2014 (in favor of the Priority Enforcement Program, which targeted detention and deportation of immigrants to those with serious criminal records). Koball's study hypothesizes that understanding the impact of Secure Communities before the Obama action will yield insights into its effect after being reinstated.

Methods and Findings

By connecting a database of state immigrant policies to U.S. Census data from the Survey of Income and Program Participation, Koball was able to analyze the impact of enforcement policies before they were loosened under Obama.

She found that in high-enforcement states in the period 2008 to 2014, immigrant households with children experienced more material hardship. Households in those states were more likely to report trouble paying their mortgages, rent, and utility bills and were less likely to get needed medical care.[11] "These policies affect 5.3 million children living with an undocumented parent, including 4.5 million U.S.-citizen children," Koball reports. The impact is felt not only by families headed by undocumented parents, but also by legal immigrant households who are not actually the target of the policies. Moreover, aggressive enforcement did not seem to financially benefit U.S.-citizen households.

> *While policies promoting immigration enforcement hurt households headed by immigrant parents, they also do not help households headed by U.S.-citizen parents.*—Heather Koball

Biomarkers of Stress and Inflammation

Zooming in from Koball's analysis of national data, Airín D. Martínez takes an in-depth look at immigrants living in Arizona. The state is home to 924,900 immigrants, about 80 percent of whom are Latinx (60%) or Asian (20.9%). Almost one-quarter (about 226,000) of the state's immigrants are unauthorized.[12] (Martinez uses the term Latinx in her research to describe a multilingual, multiracial, and multinational group with descendants from the U.S. Territory of Puerto Rico, Spanish-speaking Latin American countries, or Indigenous populations in the Americas.[13])

Martínez, a medical sociologist, joined the faculty of Arizona State University in 2013, shortly after the U.S. Supreme Court ruled on the state's Support Our Law Enforcement and Safe Neighborhoods Act. Known as SB 1070, the act criminalized unauthorized status, which had previously been a civil violation.

Dubbed the "Show Me Your Papers" law, SB 1070 required law enforcement officials to ask for documents from anyone they had "reasonable suspicion" of being in the United States without authorization and to charge those failing to carry documents with a misdemeanor. The 2012 Supreme Court decision and a 2016 settlement with the plaintiffs overturned some provisions of SB 1070, but the Secure Communities program remains, enabling ICE to take custody of individuals who have been arrested for any reason. Law enforcement personnel are permitted, but not required, to stop people and ask them for documentation.

A new resident in Arizona, Martínez was alarmed at what she viewed as SB 1070's inherent racism, which she feared would lead to extensive profiling and deter both authorized and unauthorized immigrants from sending their children to school, reporting crimes, and engaging in other civic activities. Martínez decided to examine the effect of the climate of fear on the health and stress levels of immigrant families.

A Study of Stress, Immigrant Status, and Racism

Her pilot study, conducted in 2014–2015, hypothesized that racial health inequities are associated with the stress of sustained and institutional racism. She saw "an opportunity to demonstrate that there are biological consequences to institutional forms of discrimination." Another goal was to ascertain whether Latinx immigrants were willing to participate in interviews with researchers and allow them to collect saliva, which is used to measure cortisol, a biomarker for stress, and pro-inflammatory cytokines, biomarkers for chronic disease.

Methods

Martínez randomly selected Phoenix census tracts with high rates of foreign-born Latinx residents and went door to door, accompanied by a research assistant, who was also a local community member, to recruit participating families. Thirty families totaling 111 individuals agreed to be interviewed and to donate saliva. Nineteen of them were mixed-status families, comprising both unauthorized and authorized members. Average annual family earnings were less than $20,000.

Researchers interviewed adults and children in families that self-identified as Latin American origin and in which at least one parent was foreign born. They asked about general family sources of stress, their comfort with going out in public, employment status, children's school attendance, and other factors. They also measured weight, height, and hip-to-waist circumference and analyzed saliva samples.

Findings and Lessons

Both mixed-status families and families whose members are all documented feared deportation, and that fear was associated with higher levels of inflammation, which may be related to heart disease, cancer, and other conditions later in life. Families who reported more fear of deportation also had less salivary uric acid (natural waste produced when food is digested), suggesting less antioxidant protection against free radicals (molecules produced when the body breaks down food), which are associated with heart disease, cancer, and other diseases.

Fear pervaded all aspects of family life and was especially prevalent during activities as ordinary as walking in public or trying to act responsibly by reporting a crime. Applying for a driver's license was particularly likely to generate fears of deportation.

Families lived with more than fear, however. All too often, they also felt discouraged, cut off from civic engagement, and angered by their inability to work.

Immigrants report frustration and anger because they are trapped. They can't feasibly return to where they came from, they can't provide for their families, and they are unhappy that they can't participate in society as contributing citizens.—Airín D. Martínez

Stepping back to highlight lessons learned from the study, Martínez cautions that "researchers have power" and should exhibit cultural humility and work in close concert with community organizations. Offering residents something in return for their participation is an important tool (a point that Assata Richards also emphasizes in Chapter 8: "Home, the Heart of Place"). In this study, families who were participating especially wanted information about the DACA program and about available public and community services.

Another lesson is that thoughtful and relevant research captures the attention of policymakers. Heartened by the interest of Phoenix officials, Martínez began to solicit their ideas for questions to include in her surveys.

She also underscores the importance of designing research that highlights state variations in enforcement and the availability of social services, which add important and nuanced perspectives to the findings. As well, warns Martínez, "Institutional racism is a pervasive contextual factor and should be featured in all studies." (See also "A Perspective on Black Immigrants" at the end of this chapter, where Francesca Menes explores the effects of structural racism on that population.)

Promoting Resilience in Houston

With an even larger immigrant population than Arizona, the 12-county Houston metropolitan area was in 2017 home to seven million residents,[14] speaking more than 140 languages.[15] About 1.6 million of them are immigrants, divided roughly evenly among naturalized citizens, lawful permanent residents, and unauthorized residents; an additional 5 percent live in the region legally as international students or on temporary work visas.[16]

Immigrants are at the core of Houston's economy and workforce. In 2016, they contributed $124.7 billion to the area's gross domestic product, held $38.2 billion in spending power, and paid $3.5 billion in state and local taxes.[17] Almost one-third (32%) of Houston-area workers were immigrants as were about half of the region's construction workers. More than half (56%), including 41 percent of unauthorized immigrants, owned their homes.[18]

High-Enforcement Environment

Despite their essential role in Houston's vibrant culture and economy, immigrants confront policies that undermine their capacity to thrive. A 2018 federal appeals court decision largely upheld a Texas law banning sanctuary policies in the state. Local enforcement is uneven, but communities have generally complied with requests from federal authorities to detain people suspected of being unauthorized.[19]

At least partly as a result, Houston ranks first in the country for ICE transfers from local jails to detention centers and fourth for ICE arrests in the community.[20] (In a community arrest, people are picked up in the course of their daily activities.)

The region is also home to four immigration detention centers housing more than 4,000 people, or almost 10 percent of all detainees in the United States. Eight children's shelters, operated by the federal Office of Refugee Resettlement, detain more than 1,100 children who were separated from their parents or arrived in the United States alone until they can be placed with a U.S.-based family.

National Issues Become Local

Faced with aggressive immigration policies and hostile public rhetoric, local stakeholders saw an urgent need to develop a unified and proactive stance to support the region's immigrants. The Houston Immigration Legal Services Collaborative grew out of conversations among local leaders in 2013 who were trying "to figure out how we could build capacity together," recalls the collaborative's executive director, Kate Vickery.

About 50 legal, public, social service, and business organizations now participate as members, strategizing in working groups and systems-level projects to tackle topics that include access to services, supporting crime victims, and protecting asylum seekers. The collaborative also receives and regrants funds to service providers.

"We have been thinking a lot about what we can do from an advocacy and policy perspective at the local level, both city and county," says Vickery, who is a firsthand witness to the many ways in which national issues manifest themselves locally.

Building Capacity to Protect Asylum Seekers

One of the collaborative's local projects, funded by RWJF through 2020, is to strengthen the capacity of clinicians and attorneys to work with asylum seekers in building their cases and helping them advocate for themselves through the complex immigration system.

"Making the case for asylum status has grown more difficult and complex," Vickery says, referring to a federal policy put in place by former Attorney

General Jeff Sessions that limits the use of domestic or sexual violence as a basis for asylum. Forensic evaluations of asylum seekers held in detention centers are "clinical aspects of deportation defense cases, in which you have to extensively document the harm that has been done," she explains.

Recognizing that the need for these evaluations has far outstripped the number of clinicians with expertise to conduct them, the collaborative funded the development of training curricula for clinicians and guidance tools for attorneys to help them determine when forensic evaluations are needed. It also supported Texas Children's Hospital and Baylor College of Medicine to establish a monthly asylum clinic where trained clinicians can assess asylum seekers. As well, the collaborative created a range of culturally specific self-care and trauma services to address the secondary trauma experienced by service providers.

Related projects in the Houston community are designed to help foreign-born people better integrate into their new homes. For example, the Culture of Health Advancing Together (CHAT)[21] program, which was described in a 2019 *Sharing Knowledge* poster session, offers English-as-a-second language (ESL) classes, after-school instruction, computer workshops, and more to enable immigrants from Pakistan, Afghanistan, and Iraq build skills and foster a sense of community.

Houston Immigrants After Hurricane Harvey

In a city where immigrants already faced acute challenges, August 2017 brought twin crises: one, a hurricane, the other, a shift in government policy. "Harvey fell on us—50 inches of rain literally fell," says Vickery. Along with gale-force winds, the storm knocked out power lines, disabled communication systems, crippled transportation, and hampered rescue efforts. (For more about Houston's response to Hurricane Harvey, see chapter 11: "Houston Comes Together After Hurricane Harvey.")

That same week the storm hit, the federal administration rescinded DACA and removed several countries from the list of those eligible for TPS.

The combination of events created layers of trauma as policies exposing more people to deportation took effect the same week as the worst natural disaster in our region's history.—Kate Vickery

In the immediate aftermath, DHS staff became part of the security teams at emergency shelters and aid centers. While their presence provided added capacity, it also likely deterred immigrants from accepting shelter or pursuing resources for which they were eligible. Mixed-status families are eligible for Federal Emergency Management Agency (FEMA) assistance, but many were likely afraid that seeking help could result in arrest or jeopardize future applications for permanent status. This trend has been documented in at least two studies.[22]

Longer term support for recovery came in part from FEMA, which, like ICE, is part of DHS. But for many residents, establishing proof of home ownership or tenancy, a requirement of both FEMA and private recovery grants, proved a significant barrier to help. To protect their safety, mixed-status and undocumented families may have put mortgage or rental agreements in the name of a citizen who didn't actually live in the unit, which meant they couldn't establish their legitimate rights to aid.

All of that has an impact not only on the populations directly affected, but also on the communities in which they live and work. Immigrants make up the majority of the area's emergency responders and own more than half of its independently owned businesses, which provide essential goods and services throughout the region. "These are our community members and we have to mitigate against barriers that make it difficult for our residents to recover and thrive," Vickery says.

If immigrants aren't succeeding, our region is not succeeding.—Kate Vickery

To strengthen the immigrant community in the face of emergencies, the collaborative issued its Humanitarian Action Plan[23] in March 2019, with recommendations for promoting resilience. Already, it is having an effect, according to Vickery. "People are talking more about the intersection between natural disasters and immigrants in a good way," she concludes. "When we had tropical storm Imelda in September 2019, people knew to come to us for information about eligibility for relief and other resources."

A Perspective on Black Immigrants

Turning eastward from Phoenix and Houston, Francesca Menes's work in Miami on behalf of Black immigrants calls attention to a sometimes-overlooked population within the palette of rich immigrant cultures in the United States. A few data points put her work in context.

About 4.2 million Blacks living in the United States in 2016 were born elsewhere. Of that group, which represents 10% of the American Black population, about half (49%) come from the Caribbean Islands, mostly Jamaica and Haiti. Another 39 percent hail from Africa,[24] with Nigeria and Ethiopia as the main countries of origin.[25]

Black immigrants are more likely to be living here legally (84%) than immigrants as a whole (75%).[26] They are also more likely to have become U.S. citizens (58% vs. 49%) and to speak English proficiently (74% vs. 51%).[27]

While the total population of Black immigrants is somewhat less likely than the overall U.S. population to have a college or higher degree (28% vs. 31%), Black immigrants from Africa are more likely than the population as a whole to have achieved that level of education.[28] This is partly because a large share of African immigrants enter through the Diversity Immigrant Visa program, according to a 2018 report from New American Economy,[29] a group of mayors and business leaders working to raise awareness of the economic benefits of immigration reform. The Diversity Immigrant Visa Program is a lottery open to citizens of select countries and requires that applicants have a certain level of educational achievement.[30]

In 2018, Black immigrants had a lower median household income ($697 per week vs. $758 per week)[31] compared with immigrants as a whole, but they were more likely to be working (70.8% vs. 62.9%).

"What Connects Us Is Our Blackness"

Francesca Menes grew up in the Little Haiti community of Miami, the U.S.-born daughter of an immigrant who arrived in the United States unexpectedly when her local Haitian commuter boat was rerouted to Miami during a storm. Growing up with parents who were politically engaged and buoyed by her own success as a competitive high school debater, Menes earned a college degree and joined the Florida Immigrant Coalition as an AmeriCorps apprentice of Public Allies (a social justice organization that recruits and trains young leaders). When her service ended, she stayed on for eight years, advancing into a variety of senior staff positions.

Black immigrants comprise 20 percent of all Blacks living in Florida, and the city of Miami is home to the nation's largest Haitian community. South Florida is also home to Black Africans, Caribbean Islanders, and Central and South American Blacks. "We come from different places and speak different languages," Menes says. "What connects us is our Blackness, our connected history, and the conditions in our countries that caused us to migrate here."

Despite their significant presence, Black immigrants remain somewhat invisible, largely absent from academia, media, and other seats of influence. When included in policy discussions, their experiences tend to be lumped with those of other groups, creating misleading narratives of their lives. "We have dialogues about 'people of color,' but that term needs to be disaggregated," Menes argues, noting that Haitian, Jamaican, Bahamian, and other African immigrant experiences differ from those of Latino people, who represent the majority in South Florida.

There is a huge population of Black immigrants in the United States, and our stories are not told in the media, academic, or health spaces.—Francesca Menes

Menes's challenge, and her passion, is to build a movement that looks across nationalities to identify shared experiences of achievement and hardship, while acknowledging and respecting the unique character of each culture.

Structural Racism and Criminalization of Behavior

Black immigrants confront the same forms of structural racism as U.S.-born Blacks: voter suppression, high enforcement scrutiny, profiling, and discriminatory housing, employment, health care, and education policies and practices. Proposals that could deter immigrants from participating in the U.S. Census, for example, were deliberate attempts to instill fear, Menes believes, because "the Census is not just a count. It is about our existence, what the next 10 years of our lives will look like, what resources we will receive."

They have well-founded reasons to be fearful. "Black people are significantly more likely than any other population to be arrested, convicted, and imprisoned in the U.S. criminal enforcement system, the system upon which immigration enforcement increasingly relies," according to a report by the New York University/Black Alliance for Immigration Justice.[32]

Although Black immigrants comprise only 7.2 percent of noncitizens and 5.4 percent of unauthorized residents, they represented 10.6 percent of all immigrants in deportation proceedings between 2003 and 2015, the report continued.

An Action Agenda

In her work with community organizations, businesses, and city and state officials, Menes drives an agenda aimed at empowering immigrants and nonimmigrants alike to lead a movement for change. A key principle is to support people in creating their own narratives. "I am not the person who should be sharing the story of a farmworker who has to bring her children into the field because she is afraid of being arrested if she sends them to school," Menes said.

Instead, Menes helps the children tell their own stories. As part of annual advocacy days at the Florida state capitol, hundreds of immigrants take the eight-hour bus ride to Tallahassee, delivering to legislators baskets of tomatoes picked by their parents. "Why do you want to deport my mom?" they ask. "She is the one who puts food on your table."

Advice for Researchers and Funders

In the 2019 *Sharing Knowledge* conference auditorium, filled with researchers and funders, Menes spoke openly of the "nonprofit industrial complex" that she said sometimes pits communities against one another as they compete for resources, puts small bandages on big problems, and uses siloed strategies to address interconnected issues. "Learn about Black immigrants and conduct research that is relevant to them," she urged her audience, adding that funders have the power to hold people accountable when they purport to describe Black people in their work.

Research and services related to immigrants should avoid deficit-framing terms such as "at risk," asserts Menes. In that, she echoes a message that Jose Vargas conveyed in discouraging the use of the term *illegal immigrant* in the media (see chapter 1: "The Storytellers"). "When we define people these ways, we are telling them who they are. We have to speak to their aspirations and who they can be," Menes says.

A Final Word

Policymakers across the political spectrum call for immigration reform but have been unable to agree on a course of action that will lead the country forward. Lost in the angry rhetoric are the high hopes and determination of immigrants living in the United States and the evidence demonstrating their resilience and economic and social contributions.

The activists and researchers featured in this chapter offer guidance for shifting mindsets and crafting policies that will promote equity and serve the national interest. There is evidence that the American public wants that. "Despite the divisive political landscape, when area residents were asked in the privacy of their homes about immigrants' contributions to the American economy or about welcoming endangered refugees, they continue to express increasingly favorable attitudes," concluded a 2018 report of the Rice/Kinder Institute for Urban Research.[33]

Creating communities that provide equitable opportunities for everyone is a matter not only of justice, but also of practical import. Children born into immigrant families are the country's workers, taxpayers, and civic leaders. As Airín D. Martínez reminds us, "If we don't try to maintain their health now, we reduce not only their health and futures, but the civic and economic strength of our country down the road."

The Toxic Impact of Life Behind Bars

Regina Yang Chen, MUP, Senior Director, MASS Design Group

Jim Parsons, MSc, Vice President and Research Director, Vera Institute of Justice

Kempis Songster, Communicator Lead, Amistad Law Project; Co-Founder, Ubuntu Philadelphia; Founding Member, Right 2 Redemption and Coalition to Abolish Death by Incarceration

Homer Venters, MD, MS, Author of Life and Death in Rikers Island; former Chief Medical Officer, New York City Correctional Health Services

Sara Wakefield, PhD, MS, Associate Professor, School of Criminal Justice, Rutgers University

The United States confines a higher percentage of its people in prisons and jails than any other country in the world and holds them longer, for similar crimes, than many developed countries.[1] While many states have reduced their prison populations over the last decade, spurred by public outcry and economic concerns, the U.S. incarceration rate continues to lead the world.

Less well known than the level of incarceration is its shockingly toxic impact on every aspect of a person's health and well-being. The potent interaction of prison and health is suggested by findings in a 2016 analysis by sociologist Christopher Wildeman, PhD, that life expectancy is reduced by two years for every year a person is confined.[2] The hazards of the environment were much more recently foregrounded by COVID-19, which by late June 2020 had infected almost 50,000 people in state and federal prisons and was on a rapid upswing.[3]

That toxicity radiates from incarcerated individuals to their families and communities. A startling statistic indicates the pervasive impact throughout the U.S. population: About 45 percent of Americans have had an immediate family

Regina Yang Chen, Jim Parsons, Kempis Songster, Homer Venters, and Sara Wakefield, *The Toxic Impact of Life Behind Bars*
In: *Community Resilience*. Edited by: Alonzo L. Plough, Oxford University Press (2021). © Robert Wood Johnson Foundation.
DOI: 10.1093/oso/9780197559383.003.0006

member incarcerated, as criminologist Sara Wakefield reports further in this chapter.

The contributors unpack some key components of this damaging environment and consider what a different approach to incarceration might look like. Researcher Jim Parsons at the Vera Institute of Justice provides an overview of the health impacts of incarceration, while Sara Wakefield, a Rutgers University faculty member, offers new data on family history of incarceration and opportunities to mitigate the effects. Physician Homer Venters, formerly with the New York City Correctional Health Services, describes the lack of comprehensive health outcomes data, and designer and researcher Regina Yang Chen addresses the influence of prison design on the health and well-being of residents, staff, and the community. Finally, Kempis Songster, released from prison after serving 30 years of a life-without-parole sentence for a murder he committed at age 15, grounds the narrative in lived experience. All are united in their call to reimagine the way in which the country responds to violence and crime and defines the role of incarceration.

Portrait of Incarceration

Who Is Incarcerated?

A disproportionate share of people in America who experience the toxic environments of U.S. prisons and jails are people of color, and especially likely to be Black. Some staggering statistics paint a picture of the incarcerated population:

- **The numbers are huge.** Almost 2.3 million people are incarcerated in state and federal prisons, local jails, juvenile detention facilities, military prisons, immigration detention facilities, state psychiatric hospitals, and elsewhere.[4]
- **Race plays a significant role.** In 2017, Black people were imprisoned at nearly six times the rate of Whites and nearly double that of Hispanics.[5]
- **Most incarcerated people are admitted to jails.** While almost 600,000 people enter prisons annually, close to 11 million are admitted to jails every year.[6] (More people are held in prison on a given day—about 1.5 million compared with 600,000 in jails.[7]) These short-term and generally local facilities hold people after an arrest—either until they can make bail or until they are tried if they are unable to post bail or had it denied. Some people may also serve short (less than a year) sentences at a local jail.
- **Young people are treated differently.** Some 63,000 youth under age 18 are confined in the United States, and close to 10 percent of them are imprisoned in an adult facility.[8] Many are detained for technical probation violations or

age-related status offenses, such as truancy and running away, that adults do not face. (See chapter 7: "Addressing Trauma and Building Resilience in Children: Science and Practice," for more on the impact of incarceration for status offenses.)

What Are the Health Risks?

Risks to health in prison or jail come from every direction. At a basic level, the food quality is generally poor, and overall nutrition is made worse by residents who "self-medicate" their stress with candy, cake, cookies, and chips from the commissary. Opportunities for regular exercise can be limited. Facilities are often dirty, sometimes filthy. Living close to so many people promotes high levels of communicable diseases.

On a psychological level, people are typically imprisoned hundreds of miles or more from family and lack regular support and connections to the outside world. New prisoners often arrive with untreated or poorly treated mental health and substance use disorders that are likely to worsen in an environment where little appropriate care is available (see chapter 6: "Responding to the Opioid Epidemic"). Beyond that, the stress, trauma, and violence of life in prison or jail can generate new mental health problems.

Jails and prisons are deeply unhealthy environments.—Jim Parsons

With many prisons built on former toxic waste sites, the environment is a further threat to health. Research by independent cartographer Paige Williams found that 589 of the 1,821 federal and state prisons in the United States are located within three miles of a Superfund site, areas with air and water contamination levels dangerous to public health.[9,10] Some 134 prisons are within one mile of those sites. Residents there have high levels of respiratory, gastrointestinal, and skin problems and higher than expected levels of cancer.[11]

With the increase in severe weather resulting from climate change, incarcerated people are a completely vulnerable population about whom little or no thought has been given.[12] Few plans are in place to evacuate those incarcerated in the event of a natural disaster, representing a Damoclean danger.

When people are released from incarceration, as the vast majority eventually are, they come home bearing the physical and psychological scars of their experiences. The severe damage done to their health leads to a population-level impact on a par with other public health crises, including smoking and obesity. "It requires a similar national response," urges Vera Institute's Jim Parsons. A clearer understanding of health risks—and their impact on incarcerated people and their families and communities—is essential to craft responsive policies.

Prisons and jails are the only places where there is a constitutional right to health care. It seems cruelly ironic.—Jim Parsons

Collecting Data on Family Impact

Like much of the general population, most people in prisons and jails have some combination of parents, spouses or partners, siblings, and children. When an individual is incarcerated, these connections are disrupted, and family members are at risk for their own poor health outcomes.

The impact on children can be especially severe. At least five million children have had a residential parent in prison or jail at some time during childhood, an experience that has multiple damaging long-term implications for health and well-being.[13] A single chilling finding—paternal incarceration has been found to substantially increase the risk of infant mortality—illustrates this truth.[14]

Among other dangers to family members, communicable diseases acquired in prison or jail can be transmitted when an incarcerated person returns home. African-American women are at particular risk of HIV transmission from partners who have acquired the virus in prison, engage in high-risk behaviors after release, or lack appropriate HIV care.[15]

Despite evidence of these and other far-reaching effects, "It's incredibly hard to study with the data that we have available," says Rutgers University criminologist Sara Wakefield. "We simply don't have an infrastructure to think about family members and incarceration."

To build that framework, Wakefield and a cross-country research team led by Cornell University sociologist Christopher Wildeman asked a nationally representative sample: Have you ever had an immediate family member (parent, spouse, sibling, child) incarcerated for a night or more? They also asked about extended family members, including grandparents, aunts, uncles, and cousins. Prior to their survey, there had been no nationally representative estimates that included so many different family members.

Gathering information about individuals who had spent time in jails, as well as prisons, particularly enriched the study, since data about the impacts of jail time are especially lacking. "That is where the data infrastructure problem is worst," Wakefield notes.

Finding survey participants was difficult and expensive—"something the government should be doing but isn't," in Wakefield's view. Nonetheless, a team of English- and Spanish-speaking field staff was able to gather a credible sample, including people without internet access.

What the research team found was shocking: At some point in their lives, about 45 percent of Americans have had an immediate family member incarcerated, at least for a night. And further, while there are large racial disparities, at least 30 percent of every racial and ethnic group have had that experience. Key findings of the Family History of Incarceration Survey (FamHIS) include those in the list that follows.[16,17]

Forty-five percent of Americans have had an immediate family member incarcerated, at least for a night, at some point in their lives.—Family History of Incarceration Survey

- **Racial and ethnic disparities are clear.** Sixty-three percent of Blacks and Native Americans, 48 percent of Hispanics, 42 percent of Whites, and 34 percent of other races (mostly Asian or biracial) have had an immediate family member incarcerated. Findings for Native Americans must be interpreted with caution, however, given the small sample. "The Native American community is really understudied with respect to this problem," Wakefield stresses.
- **Fourteen percent of Americans have had an immediate family member who was incarcerated for *more* than a year.** Broken down by race, the figures are 31 percent of Blacks, 29 percent of Native Americans, 11 percent of other races, and 10 percent of Whites.
- **Sixty percent of all Americans without a high school diploma have had an immediate family member incarcerated.** That is also the case among 30 percent of college graduates.
- **As income increases, the share of people who have had an immediate family member incarcerated decreases.** Fifty-three percent of adults with annual household income under $25,000 and 33 percent of those with income more than $100,000 have that experience.
- **Incarceration of a sibling was the most common experience.** Twenty-seven percent of Americans have had a sibling incarcerated, but research on the impact is limited.
- **When extended family members are included, the numbers are even more staggering.** Sixty-four percent of all Americans, and 80 percent of Black Americans, have had an immediate or extended family member incarcerated for at least one night.

This is not a niche issue. This is not something that is inconsequential. It is ubiquitous.—Sara Wakefield

As interest in criminal justice system reform grows, Wakefield sees a broader recognition among academics that it is important to study not only criminal behavior, but also the many other ways in which a larger circle of people encounter and are affected by the criminal justice system.

Government support of large-scale data collection is essential to gathering that kind of rich data so that researchers can link and analyze multiple sources. But the significant state-by-state variation in incarceration practices makes such efforts particularly challenging. Only a handful of states are committed to allowing researchers to collect data and learn from their findings; thus, a disproportionate amount of research comes from a small number of places. "Other states won't even talk to you, let alone let you in the door," Wakefield remarks.

Measuring and Understanding the Health Risks

Although the extreme conditions within prisons and jails across the country are obvious to anyone who lives, works, or visits one, the gaps in knowledge about health risks and the system to fill those gaps are sorely lacking. In 1976, the U.S. Supreme Court ruled that denial of health care to incarcerated people was unconstitutional and established the right to health care while incarcerated.[18] Correctional health services have been established in most facilities to provide that legally required care. Yet, "we are completely in the dark about basic elements of health surveillance and public health in jails and prisons, despite the fact that they are run by and accountable to governments," laments Homer Venters, former chief medical officer of New York City's jail system. "It's a travesty."

Venters began working in correctional health services shortly after the brutal beating death by other prisoners of 18-year old Christopher Robinson in October 2008 at a New York City jail on Rikers Island. Correctional officers had allowed the prisoners into Robinson's cell. This horrific incident brought to light the extensive violence rampant at the facility.[19] As Venters began treating people in the jail, he noticed a prevalence of jaw and hand fractures indicative of the violence there, but no one understood the extent of these injuries because no surveillance system existed.

Venters and colleagues began to build an injury surveillance system to capture data more reliably and add enriching details, such as whether an injury was intentional and, if so, who caused it, where it happened, when it happened, and whether the injured person was handcuffed.

They next developed an electronic medical record so that data could be aggregated, trends recognized, and outcome predictors identified. They found, for example, that people in solitary confinement are 6.9 times more likely to harm themselves than those who do not spend time there.[20]

Venters and his team also used electronic medical records to detect racial disparities in responding to mental health problems with either treatment or punishment. Analyzing 50,000 first-time jail admissions, they found that African-American and Hispanic men were more likely to be punished for a mental health issue (e.g., placed in solitary confinement), and White men were more frequently given treatment. Specifically, African-Americans faced punishment 2.4 times more than Whites, while Hispanics were 1.6 times more likely to be punished.

Critical differences in whether a person received a mental health diagnosis during the jail intake process (a more clinical encounter) or later, after getting into trouble, also emerged from their analysis. Those who were diagnosed later were more likely to be people of color, more likely to be diagnosed with a personality or antisocial disorder, and more likely to be punished.

As a result of these analyses, Venters came to believe in "the power of the electronic medical record as a human rights tool." He began to speak out about the health risks of prison and "the disconnect between the truth of what people who are incarcerated experience and the public narrative about what's happening." While recognizing that many people arrive at prison with serious pre-existing conditions, especially behavioral health issues, Venters emphasizes that "we don't acknowledge and measure the real health risks that are conferred to them *in* prison—risk of violence, sexual abuse, death." People incarcerated in prison often will not tell medical staff the truth about their physical or mental health issues "because they don't think we can help them, or that we *will* help them even if we could."

In Venters's view, the correctional health service must take on the challenge of getting at "the truth of how each jail and prison, with its own health risk profile, is harming the people who pass through." This will require pushing back on what he called the "paramilitary structure" of the security staff and public sector policies that shape the health service. Like Wakefield, Venters calls out the public sector's reluctance to fund and develop a data collection system because he believes that federal, state, and local governments bear the responsibility for ensuring that the health risks of incarceration are measured and addressed.

It is the unique responsibility of the correctional health service to tell the truth about what's happening to the people there.—Homer Venters

The Power of Design to Heal or Hurt

Given the lack of basic data about incarceration, it is not surprising that innovation in prison design has received little public support. Yet the architecture of the buildings in which we live and work, and how their functions, people flow, and the programs they house are designed, has significant impact on health and well-being. In hospitals, for example, views of nature and access to the outdoors can improve patient recovery rates and reduce self-reported pain levels.[21]

Regina Yang Chen's firm, MASS Design Group, is a nonprofit design collective committed to building, researching, and advocating for architecture that promotes justice and human dignity. Chen is especially aware of how architecture and design relate to the prison experience and the health outcomes that result.

When we think about design that can either help or hurt, that's deeply embedded in systemic justice or injustice, and architecture that reflects society's values, there is no place like the prison that so deeply encapsulates the role of design in perpetuating these impacts.—Regina Yang Chen

Prison Design and Location Have Lasting Impact

Many design decisions in today's prisons reflect past cultural attitudes toward crime and punishment. Solitary confinement, for example, was endorsed around 1800 by the Quaker community in Pennsylvania, with the goal of providing incarcerated people with private space to reflect on their misdeeds, repent, and receive absolution. It has taken hold in contemporary facilities to punish transgressions and contain or separate incarcerated individuals, and its short- and long-term psychological effects can be devastating. In a comprehensive analysis of research on solitary confinement, University of California, Santa Cruz, social psychologist Craig W. Haney, PhD, JD, MA, notes its "well-documented adverse effects" and recommends that use of solitary confinement "be eliminated entirely for some groups of prisoners and greatly reduced for others."[22]

Other features of prison layout have evolved over time to reflect changing ideas about how best to manage a fraught environment. The "panopticon" system of prison supervision, in which cells arrayed around a central core allowed staff to observe prisoners at all times, was designed by Jeremy Bentham in the 18th century to mimic God, motivate reflection, and improve behavior. Over time, the system evolved to monitoring through closed-circuit TV, which allowed correctional officers only to respond to violence, not to prevent it. The current model is direct supervision, in which officers are located in the common areas and prison workspaces where residents spend time so that they can sense the mood and diffuse potentially violent events before they escalate.

Chen describes other design decisions in prisons and jails that have enduring effects on those who live and work there:

- **Lack of privacy**—From vast hangar-like warehouses filled with row after row of metal bunks to the solitary confinement environment, which is isolated yet always on well-lit display—the lack of privacy takes its toll.
- **Cold and hard surfaces and furniture bolted to the ground** communicate that residents are also cold, hard, and violent, a dehumanizing message that robs residents of dignity.
- **Soft finishes**, on the other hand, convey respect and pride, indicating the value of those who reside there. Where prison units incorporate such design, a sense of ownership develops, the space is better cared for, and vandalism and graffiti significantly decline. Rates of sexual violence are also reduced in facilities that have piloted this design, Chen says.
- **Providing spaces, funding, and staff for vocational training and other educational programs** increases the likelihood that formerly incarcerated people will find employment after release and avoid recidivism.

In the past 30 years, the vast majority of new prison facilities have been built in rural, primarily poor, areas where local communities are eager to draw in jobs and other economic development. These remote locations make family visits much harder, cutting off critical support to the people incarcerated there. Staff may also feel removed from their communities if they must travel long distances to work. And the impact of this isolation is felt not only in prison settings but also in the home communities of both those who are incarcerated and the prison staff.

Addressing Staff Needs

The degradation of austere prison design also has substantive negative effects on prison staff. A still-cited 1982 study found that correctional officers had an average life expectancy of 59 years, compared to a national average at the time of 75.[23] Similar findings emerged from a 2011 Florida study, which found that the life expectancy of law enforcement and correctional officers was 12 years less than that of the general Florida population (62.4 vs. 74.2 years).[24] And a 2017 study in California found that one-third of correctional officers had experienced at least one symptom of post-traumatic stress disorder and 10 percent had considered suicide.[25]

Programs that focus on empowering those who are incarcerated and strengthening their educational opportunities may not achieve their goals if they do not also address staff needs. Officers might resent prisoners who receive free college classes on site when they do not have access to the same opportunity. "For change to happen," says Chen, "It all needs to happen: program change, cultural change, and buy-in from everyone at all levels."

Design Reflects Societal Goals

In U.S. society, the goal of rehabilitation competes with the desire to punish. "We continue to punish people through design: by sensory deprivation, overstimulation, and stressful environments," says Jeffery Mansfield, the design director of the MASS Design Group and a close colleague of Chen. Mansfield observed that within the criminal justice system, and among politicians and the public, there is a perception that punishment and dignity are somehow incompatible. "The system itself starts to deprive people of their humanity, both those who are incarcerated and those who work in those facilities."

What would it look like if prisons were designed for rehabilitation and healing rather than punishment and retribution? To answer that question, Chen points to Norway's Halden Prison, in which residents wear their own clothing and cook their own food in kitchens that contain knives.[26] Staff members are present within the residents' space and develop relationships with them. The outcomes? There are substantially lower rates of violent incidents and a recidivism rate less than half that of the United States. Mansfield notes a comparable decrease in violent crime in a unit created in 2018 at Turbeville Correctional Institution in South Carolina that incorporated similar design elements.

To be truly just, design must be dignifying and beautiful and able to respond to more than bare minimum human needs, creating spaces that highlight people's humanity, dignity, self-worth, and ownership.—Regina Yang Chen

An Insider's Understanding of Prison Health

As vital as data and design theory are for improving health in prisons and jails, hearing an insider's firsthand observations carries a special kind of power. Kempis Songster served more than 30 years in prison for murder before his release in December 2017. His is a compelling story of crime, remorse, redemption, and service.

Making a Life-Changing Decision

In 1987, 15-year-old Songster left his home in Brooklyn and took a train to Philadelphia with his friend Dameon. Songster was a student at a school for gifted and talented young people, and he had a caring family and a girlfriend. His decision to run away from home, he realized after much soul-searching and reflection, was "because I was overcompensating for poor showings in areas that required courage. I wanted to prove to myself that I was not a coward or a sucker and plunge myself into the most dangerous situation possible."

That he did, going deep into a Philadelphia drug gang. After a few months this life on the edge took a terrible turn, leading him and his friend to murder a 17-year-old runaway boy.

After their arrest on charges of first-degree murder, the state of Pennsylvania determined that they should be prosecuted as adults. One year later they were tried, convicted, and sentenced to life in prison without parole—a sentence that has come to be known as "death by incarceration."

Building Resilience Behind Bars

Latching on to the autobiographies of Nelson Mandela, Malcolm X, and Mark Mathabane, the South African author who rose from a background of apartheid and poverty, and lifted by the consistent support of his extended family and prison "old heads" who took him under their wing, Songster eventually recognized that "taking another life was not tough. To be tough is to fight for justice, to fight for other people, to sacrifice and to serve communities, especially those who find themselves on the downside of destiny." He read widely, worked toward a college degree, and started programs for other prisoners. He came to be called "Ghani," an Islamic name that means "rich," which he accepted as a term of endearment.

While in prison Songster founded Ubuntu Philadelphia, a program that brings together families of people who were murdered with families of people who committed murder, people who survived violence with people who caused harm. Those who are incarcerated connect by telephone, while those who have been released meet in person for community healing and restorative justice.

In 2012, the U.S. Supreme Court ruled that mandatory sentences of life without parole for juveniles were unconstitutional, and, in 2016, it confirmed that the ruling applied to people who were already in prison serving such sentences. On December 28, 2017, Songster was released on lifetime parole and walked out of Pennsylvania's Graterford Prison. He was 45 years old.

Prison Health Up Close and Personal

Since his release Songster has joined the Amistad Law Project, a Philadelphia-based public interest law center that advocates for laws and policies that support its vision of a new approach to justice. "There's nothing I want to do more than to serve some greater cause, helping to make the world a better place," he said.

From his years in prison and reflections since release, Songster has an "inside/outside" perspective on the health effects of incarceration, which he considers to be a national crisis. "For decades I saw the impact of prisons on health, up close and personal," he recalls. "Not just on the people behind the walls, but how it touches the rest of society in an insidious and noxious way."

Songster particularly focused on mental health problems in prison, which he believes are greatly underreported. "I don't believe you can go through years of incarceration unscathed," he says, "no matter how strong you are." He notes that not everyone with a mental health problem will be open about it to prison staff, given "the role the psychologist plays in your being able to make parole."

More research is also needed on the role of mental health in mass incarceration, Songster emphasizes, "because mass incarceration is in part fueled by society's failure to adequately and appropriately address mental health issues, especially in communities of color." The lack of community-based treatment options is a particular burden.

You have people who, instead of being presided over by somebody in a Black robe, should have been seen by somebody in a White smock. Instead of being judged, they should have been diagnosed. Instead of being punished, they should have been treated.—Kempis Songster

The intersection of mass incarceration and environmental justice is another issue of personal concern to Songster. He spent time at the Fayette State Correctional Institution in Pennsylvania, which is built on a coal waste dump site. A year-long investigation by the Abolitionist Law Center found "an alarming rate of serious health problems" at that facility,[27] problems that travel back to families and communities when an incarcerated individual goes home. Building prisons on such sites communicates that "the people who are housed in these toxic death chambers are worthless and written-off," says Songster.

Of the many harmful components of life in prison, Songster believes that solitary confinement wields the greatest threat to well-being. "I've seen the glassy-eyed look like death in individuals, that autistic presence from long years in solitary confinement."

But it is the cumulative effects—the "stew and brew of all of these things"—that truly destroys physical and mental health, Songster stresses. Solitary confinement, yes, but also poor diet, isolation, distance from families, physical abuse by guards, and beatings from fellow prisoners. "It's a grim picture of all of these dynamics converging to create a toxic environment so deleterious to the health and well-being and development of the individuals on the inside."

That he survived 30 years in prison and is now able to use that experience to improve the lives of others is something Songster calls "miraculous." He credits this in large part to the family support he had throughout and to "seeds planted" during his upbringing—what he had rebelled against so long ago—that began to sprout in prison, guiding his behavior and relationships, building resilience, and fostering his innate leadership capabilities. Many others, "children like me," do not fare so well, he acknowledges.

A Final Word

Treating people who are incarcerated with dignity and attention to their full range of health needs is key to enabling them to heal, develop self-worth, and play a productive role in their families and communities on release. "The removal of freedom is the punishment," Parsons observes. "Degradation and dehumanization are not supposed to be the punishment."

> Something changes in our collective psyche that we need to be deeply concerned about when we normalize living day-to-day with these kinds of narratives.
> —Kempis Songster

Experience over many decades has shown that if the prevailing narrative communicates that "those people are different, that they're not us, that money shouldn't be spent on a facility like that, then it doesn't matter what the research says," observes Chen. (Her comments about humanizing the prison population echo those of Jose Vargas, who reframes the stories we tell about unauthorized immigrants in chapter 1: "The Storytellers.")

Thus, a cultural shift, a substantive narrative change, in how we consider violence, crime, and the restoration of individuals, families, and communities is necessary to build support for a more humane, public health approach to criminal justice. A public health perspective means considering the root causes of violence, and how those causes can be ameliorated, rather than responding with "a knee-jerk, punitive reaction to the symptom of the cause," as Parsons describes it. Songster contrasted the tools of public safety—"more police, more prisons, and harsher sentences"—with the tools of public health: "healing, restorative justice, and trauma responsiveness." The goal of ensuring that people are healthy on release and can become contributing family and community members is a public health goal.

Finally, and perhaps most importantly, "There is no healing without accountability," Songster recognizes. Accountability must come from "those of us who have left tears in the fabric of life and holes in the cosmos by things that we have done, whatever the socioeconomic and environmental circumstances behind our acts." Accountability for one's actions is not living for years in a cell. Rather it is admitting to what one did, apologizing for it, asking forgiveness, and pledging to be an agent of change. This can be the foundation of a different kind of justice system, one that will lift people up, build individual and community resilience, and benefit all people in this country, for we are all affected by the American way of justice.

> *It's not just about those millions behind the walls, it's also about what this does to the rest of the 320 million of us.*—Kempis Songster

SECTION II

SYSTEMIC BARRIERS
TO RESILIENCE

We explored the role of narrative and the value of an inclusive approach to gathering stories and data in the opening part of this book. This framing helps to personalize our shared social and policy challenges. In this next part, we go deeper into those challenges as they influence the capacity for resilience.

When we think about what it means for individuals, families, and communities to be resilient, certain images come to mind. There's a community working together to withstand and recover from the devastation of a wildfire, coastal flooding, or a storm or to speak out boldly against racism. There's a family insisting that local government officials monitor their air and water quality after a nearby toxic chemical spill. There's an individual cobbling together a package of social and health services in a deeply fragmented system. And as an uncertain world confronts an unpredictable pandemic, health care workers on the front lines epitomize resilience as they tirelessly show up to care for COVID-19 patients.

But for some, the capacity to show resilience is limited not by a lack of personal strength but by inequitable or exclusionary policies, practices, and procedures. This reality highlights "issues of social vulnerability and differential access to power, knowledge, and resources" that inform the concept of equitable resilience.[1] As our understanding of what it takes to build a Culture of Health deepens, new images emerge of people who face systemic barriers to resilience. There's the immigrant, living in fear of a knock on the door; the incarcerated individual in an environment characterized by poor-quality health care; people with opioid use disorders in rural areas who cannot access proven treatments; teenage girls whose lives and futures are defined by trauma and abuse; and families who confront discrimination as they seek the sanctuary of a place called home.

The three chapters in this section unfold with sometimes-stark portraits of the inequities and discrimination that are rooted in history but loom as large today as ever before. There are also glimmers of hope, with portraits of programs that are making a difference.

Chapter 6, "Responding to the Opioid Epidemic," describes efforts to address opioid use disorders in two distinct environments—correctional settings and rural areas. Pockets of progress in this national health crisis not only provide examples of hope, but also underscore the sobering reality that proven treatment methods are not being extended to those who need them most. The chapter explains why barriers to resilience exist and why progress sometimes stalls.

Chapter 7, "Addressing Trauma and Building Resilience in Children: Science and Practice," is a poignant, research based look at the impact of early adversity and trauma and the buffers that can nurture resiliency. The chapter focuses on the unique experiences of girls, with a glimpse into the impact of childhood maltreatment on brain development and the potential for recovery and resilience in later life. It also looks at the power of texting during a crisis, a community-through-technology tool that resonates remarkably well in the era of the coronavirus pandemic.

This section ends with chapter 8, "Home, the Heart of Place," which underscores the continuing assault of racial inequities, discriminatory lending practices, and geographic disparities around housing. Through personal stories and exhaustive research, contributors look at redlining and racism, the health consequences of substandard housing, the affordability crisis, and the relationship between home ownership and neighborhood well-being. A look at Houston's Third Ward explains why the value of a neighborhood is captured not only in a real estate closing statement, but also in the eyes of its residents. A key portal to a Culture of Health, home is so much more than just four walls.

Responding to the Opioid Epidemic

Elizabeth Connolly, MS, Director, Substance Use Prevention and Treatment Initiative, Pew Charitable Trusts

John Gale, MS, Senior Research Associate, Maine Rural Health Research Center, Muskie School of Public Service, University of Southern Maine

Throughout 2019, media headlines seemingly surfaced daily to describe a country confronting an opioid epidemic that was devastating individuals, families, and communities nationwide:

> *The Opioid Crisis Is a National Emergency . . . How Much Money Will It Take to Undo the Damage from Opioids? . . . Opioids Are an Equal-Opportunity Killer . . . Opioid Epidemic Disproportionately Affects Rural Communities . . . Washington Tackles Opioid Use Disorder in Its Jails . . . Making Drug Companies Pay for the Opioid Epidemic*

According to the Office of the Assistant Secretary for Health, over 11 million people misuse opioid pain relievers and heroin every year, and another two million develop a full-blown opioid use disorder, characterized by serious impairment or distress.

Despite such ominous reports, 2019 also produced some encouraging news. Consider:

- Nationwide, prescriptions for opioids peaked at 255 million in 2012 and then steadily declined for the next five years, reaching a 10-year low of 191 million in 2017, the latest year for which statistics are available.[2]
- Three decades of escalating deaths from drug overdoses appeared to come to an end. According to the Centers for Disease Control and Prevention (CDC), mortality estimates from 2017 through February 2019 suggested a

Elizabeth Connolly and John Gale, *Responding to the Opioid Epidemic* In: *Community Resilience*. Edited by: Alonzo L. Plough, Oxford University Press (2021). © Robert Wood Johnson Foundation. DOI: 10.1093/oso/9780197559383.003.0007

5 percent drop in overdose deaths in the United States,[3] representing the first yearly decline since 1990.[4]

- Drug manufacturers and distributors faced a flurry of lawsuits about their responsibility in fostering the crisis, although they continued to deny wrongdoing for promoting opioid use. While litigation is still ongoing in 2020, individual companies have already agreed to multiple multibillion-dollar settlements over the next two decades to address opioid addiction.[5]

- Throughout the country, innovative medication-assisted treatment (MAT) programs and evidence-based community efforts have emerged to help individuals overcome opioid addiction and reduce the stigma associated with it. What experts call a "conclusive body of evidence" now shows that MAT is the most effective way to treat opioid use disorder.

Opioid use disorder is a complex, relapsing brain disease for which there is effective treatment. This devastating loss of life is preventable.—Elizabeth Connolly

This chapter examines the complex disease of opioid use disorder and the barriers that exist within the very system designed to help. It also highlights some promising pockets of progress, focusing especially on two environments hit hard by opioid addiction: correctional settings and rural areas.

Elizabeth Connolly of the Pew Charitable Trusts argues persuasively that MAT improves outcomes for incarcerated individuals with opioid use disorders after they are released and presents examples of successful MAT programs in Massachusetts and Colorado. John Gale, a researcher at the Maine Rural Health Research Center, explains the multiple, complex factors that contribute to the prevalence of opioid addiction among rural populations, shedding light on why rural communities are disproportionately impacted by this epidemic. He then describes a set of evidence-based models being used to tackle opioid addiction in rural communities, with pockets of progress reported. The chapter concludes with a look at why more progress has not been made.

Stark Numbers, Human Tragedy, and a Bit of Hope

Decades of scientific research show that addiction is a chronic disease of the brain. Scientists know that prolonged use of prescription opioids, heroin, or other illicit opioids causes life-threatening and long-lasting effects that can lead to opioid tolerance, physical dependence, and addiction.[6] The terms *substance use disorder* and *opioid use disorder* are sometimes used interchangeably in reports and in the media, but substance use disorder is an umbrella term that can also include alcohol, marijuana, nicotine, heroin, and other addictive substances; opioid use disorder is the subset of substance use disorder in which opioids are the primary drug being misused. The opioid focus is closely tied to the increased use of prescription pain treatment that began nearly 30 years ago.[7]

Though the abuse of prescription opioids containing oxycodone has been a concern in the United States since the 1960s, experts at the CDC frame the most recent opioid crisis as having three distinct waves. "The first wave began in the 1990s with the increased prescribing of opioids. The second wave began in 2010, with rapid increases in overdose deaths involving heroin. The third wave began in 2013, with significant increases in overdose deaths involving synthetic opioids—particularly those involving illicitly manufactured fentanyl."[8]

After the first wave, the death-by-overdose epidemic escalated until it was identified as the primary cause of the drop in life expectancy from 2015 through 2018, a pattern not documented in the United States since World War II.[9] In stark numbers, from 1999 to 2017 more than 700,000 people in the United States died from a drug overdose. In 2017 alone, the most recent year for which data are available, that figure was 70,200, with 68 percent or 47,736 of these deaths involving an opioid—six times more than in 1999.[10]

The bottom line? Even with a recent decline, an average of 130 Americans still die every day from an opioid overdose.[11] That's five people who die every hour or one every 11 minutes.

The epidemic is about not only statistics, but also human tragedy. The indiscriminate reach of the crisis—from rural communities to urban street corners, from prison cells to Native American homelands, from Wall Street corridors to homeless shelters—results in the deaths of people like Rachel Bandman, the 19-year-old University of South Carolina student who was battling depression; Elisa Serna, 24, who died in a San Diego County jail; Steve Rummler, a 43-year-old musician from Minnesota who suffered a back injury as an adult, became addicted to pain medication, and relapsed after completing a 28-day addiction treatment program; District Court Judge Tom Jarrell, 56, of Guilford County, N.C., found dead in his home of a fentanyl and heroin overdose; and Marisa Gyorr, who grew up on a farm in rural Illinois and died at the age of 20.[12]

Ashley McAuliffe of Hayden, Colorado, is not one of the opioid epidemic's five-deaths-every-hour statistic. Like 63 percent of those with an opioid use disorder,[13] McAuliffe first used prescription painkillers for pain, in her case when she was a teenager recovering from ski and snowboarding injuries. In 2018, after her second overdose, McAuliffe turned for help to a newly available MAT program, and the treatment has been working. Two years later, she was raising a family and working as a manager of an upscale grocery store near her home.

Without MAT, she told her local newspaper, her recovery "would have been impossible."[14]

McAuliffe's story reflects two facts about addiction: It is a disease, and it can be treated.

People with OUD [opioid use disorder] have a chronic disease that warrants long-term medical management, like insulin for diabetes or blood pressure medication for hypertension.—National Academies of Sciences, Engineering, and Medicine, Consensus Study[15]

The research shows clearly that methadone, buprenorphine, and naltrexone all help reduce opioid cravings and sharply reduce the risks of overdose and death.[16] Methadone and buprenorphine also alleviate withdrawal symptoms. Coupled with behavioral therapy and counseling—the complementary therapies that comprise the assistance in "medication-assisted treatment"—these three drugs are considered the gold standard for treating opioid use disorder.

Opioids and Incarceration

The opioid epidemic and substance use disorder are inextricably associated with incarcerated individuals in correctional settings. (Drugs, however, are far from the only health challenges facing incarcerated populations as Chapter 5: "The Toxic Impact of Life Behind Bars" amply demonstrates.) According to Prison Policy Initiative, males, Blacks, and Latinos "are disproportionately incarcerated" and make up most of the incarcerated populations.[17] When it comes to statistics on incarceration and substance use, consider the following:

- At least one in five incarcerated individuals is imprisoned on drug charges.[18]
- More than half (58 percent) of individuals incarcerated in state prisons and almost two-thirds (63 percent) of individuals who have been sentenced to jail terms met the medical criteria for substance use disorder—compared to 5 percent of the general adult population.[19] But only 22 percent of incarcerated individuals with a substance use disorder have participated in a treatment program, and most of those programs offer counseling and promote abstinence from drugs but provide no medications.[20]
- At least one-quarter of the people in U.S. prisons and jails are addicted to opioids.[21] But only 5 percent of people with opioid use disorder in jail and prison settings received medication for opioid use disorder, according to a recent National Academies of Science study.[22]

Justice-involved individuals are especially vulnerable to overdose and dying after their incarceration ends. "Treatment Behind Bars," a study by Stateline, an initiative of the Pew Charitable Trusts, found that incarcerated individuals who are released from prisons and jails "rejoin their communities with dangerously reduced tolerance and nothing to blunt their drug cravings, making them highly susceptible to a deadly overdose."[23]

A recent study in North Carolina reached a similar conclusion with its finding that former inmates were 40 times more likely to die of an opioid overdose in the first two weeks after being released than someone in the general population.[24]

> *We can all agree that people who are justice-involved are an underserved population with a number of health disparities and health inequities, including substance use disorders.*—Elizabeth Connolly

The Case for MAT

Elizabeth Connolly developed an interest in justice-involved populations during her long career in human services for the state of New Jersey. As then-Governor Chris Christie was making substance use, prevention, and treatment the focus of his agenda, Connolly was commissioner of human services.

After nearly 30 years in state government, Connolly joined Pew Charitable Trusts in 2018 to "focus on something that had become a passion of mine— substance use disorder treatment, prevention, and recovery."

Connolly argues that "individuals who receive MAT while incarcerated saw better post-incarceration outcomes than those who did not." In one study, for example, MAT users had longer times to re-arrest after being released compared to individuals who were only offered detoxification while in prison and jails.[25]

The value of medication while incarcerated was also confirmed in a Rhode Island study, where individuals maintained on methadone behind bars were twice as likely to receive treatment following their release and almost two-thirds less likely to die from an opioid overdose. And in a Maryland study, individuals who received buprenorphine were more likely to continue treatment following their release than those who received counseling only. Still other research showed that people who receive MAT are less likely to die of overdose, use illicit opioids, or contract infectious diseases, such as HIV and hepatitis C, compared to nonmedication approaches.

Connolly noted that most of the MAT studies on incarcerated individuals involved men, who make up the vast majority of incarcerated people. But she emphasized that incarcerated women who are pregnant "are a priority for MAT" to ensure that they are not detoxing while pregnant and recent statistics on incarcerated women suggest broader needs for MAT. According to a 2019 book,

Getting Wrecked: Women, Incarceration, and the American Opioid Crisis, death from prescription opioid overdose increased nearly 500 percent among women since 1999 (compared with a 200 percent rise among men); at the same time, the rate at which women are incarcerated has grown twice as fast as that of men.[26]

Connolly argues that providing treatment during incarceration also offers significant benefits to communities and families after release, an assertion supported by the National Institute on Drug Abuse: "A growing number of studies show the benefits of initiating medication treatment (methadone, buprenorphine, or naltrexone) before release from jail or prison. The benefits include reduced drug use and risk of overdose death, as well as reduced risk of infectious disease transmission and improved clinical outcomes when infected with HIV."[27]

And finally, Connolly's support of MAT includes an economic argument. "MAT is shown to reduce emergency and hospitalization costs, people can go back to work, families are reunited, child welfare spending decreases, and drug-related crimes drop. So if you need to make the economic case, you can go there."

Pockets of Progress in Correctional Settings

To better illustrate the benefits of MAT, Connolly described three pockets of progress in the states.

Middlesex County, Massachusetts

Middlesex County, Mass., is the most populous county in New England, with nearly 1.6 million residents. Between 2010 and 2016, opioid-related overdoses in the county increased by over 300 percent, and by 2016 represented 10 percent of all fatal opioid-related overdoses in Massachusetts, one of the states hit hardest by the opioid crisis. Also reflecting the scope of the challenge, nearly 40 percent of the county's incarcerated population required immediate drug or alcohol detoxification when they were detained, with 73 percent specifically requiring opioid detoxification.[28]

In response to the escalating epidemic, the Middlesex Sheriff's Office launched the Medication Assisted Treatment and Directed Opioid Recovery (MATADOR) program in 2015 with the triple goal of saving lives, reducing crime, and improving public health. The pilot framed incarceration as an opportunity to create a pathway to success following release.

This voluntary program helps individuals in jail avoid relapse into addiction—and potentially related criminal activity—by combining MAT and six months of postrelease recovery and community support from the staff. (Originally, the pilot used naltrexone alone, but it was expanded in September 2019 to offer methadone and buprenorphine as well.) Data examining drug relapse, overdose, and recidivism are being collected to inform program performance.

By April 2018, MATADOR had enrolled more than 337 people in custody; among those who have completed the program, 82 percent have not recidivated. Impressed by its success, the Massachusetts legislature mandated a four-year project that expands the pilot program to a total of seven jails.

Denver, Colorado

Citing a high rate of overdose deaths in this city of 705,000—and the fact that three-quarters of individuals are addicted to drugs or alcohol at the time they are incarcerated—Denver Health, the main health care system providing services to incarcerated individuals, worked in 2018 with the Denver Sheriff's Department to expand its MAT program inside the Denver County Jail. Anyone entering the jail on methadone would be allowed to continue using it; others could be evaluated and receive the appropriate MAT on request while incarcerated. The program also provided counseling and other services postrelease and continued the Sheriff's Department practice of providing methadone to inmates.

Based on the success of the Denver program, the Colorado legislature required jails receiving state money for drug treatment programs to include MAT for any incarcerated individual who requests it, reducing prior authorization barriers. Previously, notes Connolly, only five of the state's 57 jails used state funds to provide addiction medications, choosing instead to pay for counseling and housing assistance on release. The new law has become a cornerstone in Colorado's efforts to end its opioid epidemic.[29]

Denver County's "Opioid Response Strategic Plan for 2018–2023" also made improved treatment for substance use disorder and MAT participation in jails a priority. In addition to community treatment on demand and access to safe syringes, the plan identifies the goals of scaling up jail-to-community MAT programs; increasing the number of people who participate in MAT while in jail; and increasing the number of previously incarcerated individuals maintained on MAT for three months after reentry into the community.[30]

Atlantic County, New Jersey

When she worked for the state of New Jersey, Connolly helped launch a decidedly mobile pocket of progress: a van that offers methadone or buprenorphine to people with opioid addiction in Atlantic County, a diverse jurisdiction that includes Atlantic City and smaller beach towns, as well some inland rural municipalities. When the warden of the county's only jail recognized the need for better access to drug treatment, Connolly arranged to extend the state's methadone van program to the Atlantic County jail. (At the time, New Jersey was part of a federal pilot to provide mobile methadone services. Although program funding for new vans has since been frozen, states where vans were already in use continue to use them.)

Connolly stresses that progress against addiction in rural communities often depends on having a "champion" to promote the cause. In the case of Atlantic County, a county judge and the county jail warden assumed that mantle.

Folks who are champions of opioid addiction recovery come to it with passion. And that's needed. It's a long road—and it is hard.—Elizabeth Connolly

Rural Communities and Opioids

The growth in the use of heroin, prescription opioids, and methamphetamines has hit rural communities disproportionately, resulting in what one Robert Wood Johnson Foundation (RWJF) study called a "particularly daunting impact."[31] According to recent research:

- Fourteen of the 15 counties with the highest opioid prescription rates in the country are designated as rural.[32] People living in rural areas have an 87 percent higher chance of receiving an opioid prescription compared to those in metropolitan areas, leading to far greater rates of dependency and opioid use disorders.[33]
- The opioid overdose death rate in rural areas surpassed that in urban areas in 2015, increasing by 325 percent between 1999 and 2015.[34] By 2017, according to a study in RWJF's "Rural Health and Well-Being" initiative, opioid-related overdose deaths were 45 percent higher in rural communities than in metro-area counties.[35]
- Rural youth are 35 percent more likely to have misused prescription opioids in the past year, compared to their urban peers. As in incarceration settings, the consequences of their greater opioid use include not only more overdose deaths but also increased exposure to HIV and hepatitis C.[36]

It has affected the whole population, but it's been a uniquely rural problem going back to the 90s when OxyContin was first available and known as "Hillbilly Heroin." It's a complex problem. And now it seems the "rural" problem looks a lot like most of the country.—John Gale

The Distinctive Character of Rural Challenges

John Gale likes to claim that his upbringing makes him uniquely qualified to conduct research at the Maine Rural Health Research Center. "I grew up in a rural community in Maine," he says, laughing, "and I've shoveled manure and I've baled hay. I also spent many years working with physicians and providers in Maine."

The emphasis of RWJF on rural health and leadership aligns with Gale's assertion. "The best rural leadership comes from within rural communities," the foundation recently wrote in one of its fact sheets. "Rural leaders are taking on—and finding innovative solutions for—some of our country's most significant challenges, including the opioid crisis."[37]

Gale is especially attuned to the drivers of addiction in rural Maine, which is among the top 10 states with the highest rates of opioid-related overdose deaths.[38] As in other parts of rural America, local people suffer from a variety of health and socioeconomic disparities that contribute to addiction: isolation and hopelessness; lower education rates; higher rates of poverty; a greater sense of stigma; fewer opportunities for employment; higher rates of chronic illness; and inadequate insurance, which restricts the ability to seek medical help, making it more tempting to turn instead to illicit painkillers.

"I remember interviewing a fisherman who had a terrible injury from catching his hand in a winch," Gale recalls. "He couldn't afford OxyContin prescriptions, because he didn't have health insurance and the price of pills was so high. So he resorted to buying heroin to manage his pain."

We're not going to fix this by just controlling the flow and prescriptions of OxyContin and other synthetic opioids. We're not going to fix it by tamping down on heroin. We have to do both, of course, but we have to begin to look at the drivers behind this crisis.—John Gale

Gale pointed to several distinctive features of rural areas. One is that recovery programs imported from elsewhere are often viewed with suspicion. To engage local leaders, he cautions, community-based programs must be sensitive to local culture, religion, and ethnic issues. And these programs must support sober living, with safeguards in place against relapse, such as enhancing social supports, providing vocational opportunities, and reducing the stigma associated with treatment. "Everybody knows your business in rural towns," he comments, acknowledging the difficulty of remaining anonymous.

Most opioid users in small towns and communities have burned a few bridges. They have taken advantage of their families. Law enforcement officials know who they are. And if they can't go back and find some path to the future, treatment will be a revolving door. Most people take four to five years of being in and out of remission before they get on the right track. Less than 50 percent admitted to treatment complete it.—John Gale

Gale stresses that rural populations deserve the same access to treatment services as urban populations—but often don't get them. Because they are chronically medically underserved, seeing a doctor or filling a prescription often requires considerable travel. Gale is an advocate for tools that integrate technology-driven "telemedicine" or "telehealth" programs into clinical care, allowing physicians to provide counseling remotely and addressing the barriers of distance and lack of resources.

Pockets of Progress in Rural Settings

When it comes to fighting rural addiction, Gale points to several evidence-based models that are having some success. A brief description of these models follows, with a few examples of programs in each category.

Community Organizing Models

Community organizing models use active participation from the community to create strategies for addressing opioid addiction. One example is Project Lazarus, a community-based program that encourages physicians to prescribe naloxone, the antidote for opioid overdose, to patients at highest risk. It also promotes community education to spread the message that overdose deaths are preventable, and that all communities are responsible for the health of their own citizens. Project Lazarus is in place throughout North Carolina and has influenced programs in Michigan, Ohio, Pennsylvania, and Wisconsin.[39]

Another initiative with roots in local organizing is Project Vision in Rutland, Vermont, which engages residents to approach the rural community's substance use problems in creative ways. The interventions don't always get at root causes, but they can reduce the supply of opioids in a neighborhood under siege. For example, after being alerted by the community to a home where known dealers are living, police park a brightly colored van there and "lo and behold, the drug dealers move on," says Gale. "You aren't solving the problem, but you are helping deter the problem in your community, which is the only thing the local police can hope to do."

Prevention Models

Prevention models limit access to prescription opioids and can help reduce supply and discourage or delay onset of substance use disorders. These cost-effective approaches can be targeted to specific populations, such as children, adolescents, young adults, or pain patients. Strategies include hospital prevention plans to reduce the level of opioid prescribing, alternative pain-management strategies, and opportunities to dispose of unneeded medications.

For instance, the Midcoast Maine Prescription Opioid Reduction Program sought to reduce the number of emergency department dental patients abusing opioid prescriptions in rural southeastern Maine. After new prescription protocol guidelines were put into place at two rural hospitals that serve roughly 17,000 patients a year, the rate of opioid prescription dropped nearly 20 percent, and dental pain emergency department visits fell from 26 to 21 per 1,000.[40] Gale notes that emergency departments all over the country, recognizing that they are a frequent target for those seeking opioids, have embraced the concept of an "oxy-free zone" and limited opioid prescriptions.

Another substance abuse prevention effort is keepin' It REAL (an acronym for Refuse, Explain, Avoid, and Leave), a middle school–based program adapted specifically for rural cultures. Keepin' It REAL uses personal stories of adolescent drug experiences, along with interactive lessons and other videos, to help students learn to say no to drugs. In a program designed for rural areas in Pennsylvania and Ohio, an evaluation showed that students used fewer substances and found them less personally acceptable.[41]

Hospital-Based Treatment Program Models

Models of hospital-based treatment programs include everything from MAT programs at Maine's Bridgton Hospital to expanding local pain management services at Salem Township Hospital, a rural hospital about an hour from Marion, Illinois. Twice a month, a pain specialist from Marion sees patients in Salem, where patients continuing with opioids must agree to regular drug tests and not ask for early refills. Over three to four months, the hospital reported that only three out of 56 patients chose to stick with opioids, says Gale.

Why Pockets of Progress Are Too Few

Given the pockets of progress described here—and the scientific consensus that MAT is the gold standard to treat opioid use disorder—the questions seem obvious. Why aren't more people with opioid use disorder getting the help they need? Why aren't we more successful at fighting this epidemic?

The answer, according to experts, is actually quite shocking: The tools that have proven capable of fighting this epidemic are not being widely used. "Most people who could benefit from medication-based treatment for opioid use disorder do not receive it," states a National Academies report flatly.[42] The reasons to explain why are many and complex.

Medication and Treatment Tools Are Not Being Used

According to Elizabeth Connolly, only one in nine Americans with a substance use disorder, and only one in four with an opioid use disorder, received any kind of treatment in 2017. Although almost 14,000 facilities across the country provided some kind of substance use treatment in 2018, fewer than half offered MAT, and only 3 percent of those made all three approved medications available.

Among prison populations, the statistics are even bleaker. Fewer than 1 percent of the more than 5,000 U.S. prisons and jails allow access to the medications approved to treat addiction, even though 63 percent of people in jails met the medical criteria for substance use disorder (which excludes alcohol).[43] Increasingly, these limitations are being challenged in court.

> *There is no scientific evidence that justifies withholding medications for opioid use disorder patients in any setting. . . . To withhold treatment or deny services under these circumstances is unethical.*—National Academies[44]

Major Barriers to Treatment

According to the National Academies, the opioid crisis cannot be adequately addressed until experts confront the major barriers to widespread use and acceptance of effective medications. These barriers include the following[45]:

- **The misunderstanding and stigma directed at drug addiction, individuals with opioid use disorder, and the medications to treat it.** Because methadone and buprenorphine are both forms of opioids, many in the law enforcement and medical fields see them as trading one addictive drug for another. As well, many communities adopt a "not in my backyard" approach to drug treatment clinics.

> *Criminal justice stigma and stigma around MAT is pervasive. "Oh, you're just replacing one drug with another." "They brought this on themselves." "They are not worthy of treatment in jail." I was in a meeting several months back and someone suggested we just let everybody die. That was an awful day.*—Elizabeth Connolly

- **Inadequate education and training of the professionals responsible for working with people with opioid use disorder,** including treatment providers and law enforcement and other criminal justice personnel.

Despite a history of research showing sustained benefits from MAT, the Stateline report on treatment behind bars notes that opposition often comes from within prison walls. "Standing in the way are sheriffs and other prison officials, who argue that allowing treatment inside prisons with methadone or buprenorphine will lead to the drugs being diverted within the prison and possibly to illicit street markets," states the report.[46]

This barrier—and the stigma shift from drug use to the treatments associated with it—is not lost on those who study the issue.

The scientific understanding of OUD differs from public perception of the disorder, which is colored by the misconception of addiction as simply a moral failing. The social stigma that has long been directed at those who use drugs has now spread to the medications used to treat OUD.—National Academies[47]

Gale points out that these same barriers make it challenging to provide treatment and MAT services in rural areas. One issue, he says, "is the maldistribution of specialty providers, including those with Medicaid waivers to prescribe buprenorphine, which disadvantages rural areas."

Too, even those rural physicians, nurse practitioners, and physician assistants who are permitted to prescribe buprenorphine often don't do so, given the stigma of treating drug users or "addicts," says Gale, echoing the same issue faced by prison officials. "Many more prescribers receive waivers than incorporate them into their practices. This problem is a particular challenge in rural areas."

One of the best ways to fight this stigma in rural areas, notes Gale, is the hub-and-spoke model for MAT that has been adopted in Vermont. The hubs (regional specialty treatment centers) provide comprehensive care management and referrals to the spokes (community physicians and collaborating health and addiction professionals), who dispense buprenorphine, monitor adherence to treatment, and coordinate access to recovery supports.[48]

- **Current policies around the use of naltrexone, methadone, and buprenorphine to treat opioid addiction and the fragmented system of paying for care.** The National Academies report notes that "access varies among different treatment settings. For those entering the criminal justice system, MAT is often withheld or provided on a limited basis. Most residential treatment facilities do not offer medications and, if they do, they rarely offer all three medications. Expanding access through settings such as community health centers and mobile medication units would save lives and build the capacity to make real progress against the epidemic."[49]

In particular, Medicaid's refusal to pay for treatment inside jails is a significant barrier. Connolly, Gale, and countless others have urged Congress to support states in expanding opioid use disorder treatment in all settings.

Recognizing that Medicaid is the largest source of coverage and funding for substance use prevention and treatment nationally, RWJF has championed Medicaid expansion on several levels, including expanding MAT for use outside designated opioid treatment programs and increasing the number of patients that qualified providers can serve.[50] In a 2019 health policy brief, RWJF noted, "State Medicaid programs are the bedrock of state efforts to fight the still-raging opioid epidemic, and the substance use crisis overall . . . and are becoming models for all-payer efforts to combat addiction."

A Final Word

At the beginning of 2018, the Aspen Health Strategy Group, an initiative of the Aspen Institute's Health, Medicine, and Society program, released a report called "Confronting Our Nation's Opioid Crisis," which was supported in part by RWJF. Calling it one of the top health issues facing our country, the report notes the opioid epidemic is an equal opportunity crisis that "has hit people across the country of every race and ethnicity, regardless of where they live," and that prevalence levels in urban areas now match those in rural regions.[51]

No matter where the crisis is located, even the most encouraging news about opioid use carries a long shadow. By late 2019, researchers took a further look into the data suggesting that the crisis had peaked and discovered some ominous news. While the total number of opioid prescriptions had dropped, the length of time covered by prescriptions has gotten longer, which means the same number of pills, or even more of them, can be prescribed. Moreover, the decline in drug overdose deaths that was first reported in mid-2019 reflected a dip associated with prescription opioids—but fatal overdoses involving fentanyl, methamphetamine, and other drugs continued to rise.[52]

In particular, methamphetamine overdoses in rural areas have surged; according to the CDC, roughly 14,000 cocaine users and 10,000 meth users died in the United States in 2017, an increase of more than a third compared with 2016 and triple the number in 2012.[53] Gale notes that "disturbing reports" show that drug overdose deaths in Maine and other rural states appear to be rising again after a slight decline in 2018, highlighting the continuing challenge.[54]

"The substance use problem is like a big balloon," he concludes. "If you reduce access to one type of drug by reducing supply through prescribing guidelines or law enforcement programs, it looks like you've made progress. But unless you address the underlying drivers of substance use through prevention and treatment programs, another area will just pop out as individuals substitute other drugs to cope with their substance use disorders."

Addressing Trauma and Building Resilience in Children

Science and Practice

Angela Diaz, MD, PhD, MPH, Jean C. and James W. Crystal Professor, Department of Pediatrics and Department of Environmental Medicine and Public Health, Icahn School of Medicine at Mount Sinai; Director, Mount Sinai Adolescent Health Center

Rebecca Epstein, JD, Executive Director, Georgetown Law Center on Poverty and Inequality

Bob Filbin, MA, Chief Data Scientist and Co-Founder, Crisis Text Line

Amanda Sheffield Morris, PhD, Regents Professor and George Kaiser Family Foundation Endowed Chair in Child Development; Human Development and Family Science, Oklahoma State University

Martin Teicher, MD, PhD, Director, Developmental Biopsychiatry Research Program, McLean Hospital, and Associate Professor of Psychiatry, Harvard Medical School

Research over the past two decades reveals that the early experience of adversity is closely connected to a greater likelihood of engaging in risky behaviors and to negative health and well-being outcomes. Advances in neuroscience have identified the mostly irreversible changes in the developing brain that occur when a young person is maltreated or witnesses violence. By perhaps unsurprising

Angela Diaz, Rebecca Epstein, Bob Filbin, Amanda Sheffield Morris, and Martin Teicher, *Addressing Trauma and Building Resilience in Children* In: *Community Resilience*. Edited by: Alonzo L. Plough, Oxford University Press (2021).
© Robert Wood Johnson Foundation. DOI: 10.1093/oso/9780197559383.003.0008

contrast, we have also learned that positive and supportive experiences can help youth build the lasting personal resilience essential to confronting life's challenges.

The potential lifelong consequences of adversity and trauma among girls differ from those of boys. And those consequences can be severe, as the previous chapter documents in the rising rates of incarceration and growing numbers of deaths from prescription opioid addiction among women (see chapter 6: "Responding to the Opioid Epidemic").

To dive further into the mechanisms by which long-term adversity and trauma harm and what that reveals about resilience, this chapter opens with a dip into scientific research. Although biology is not generally central to the Robert Wood Johnson Foundation's (RWJF's) *Sharing Knowledge* conferences, the cutting-edge science here provides essential context for understanding the enduring damage that occurs.

After a research overview, Harvard Medical School psychiatrist and neuroscientist Martin Teicher explains how childhood maltreatment affects the developing brain and what that means for resilience and recovery. Developmental psychologist Amanda Sheffield Morris from Oklahoma State University then describes a new model to mitigate the effects of trauma.

In the second section of the chapter, examples from practice offer deeper insights into the unique experiences of girls, their potential for resilience, and the power of mitigation. Mount Sinai Adolescent Health Center physician Angela Diaz presents troubling data about the extent of sexual abuse among girls, while attorney and advocate Rebecca Epstein of Georgetown Law Center on Poverty and Inequality argues for rethinking the ways in which girls—especially girls of color—are victimized by systems that should be on their side.

The chapter closes with an example of using technology to confront trauma. Bob Filbin, the co-founder of the Crisis Text Line, describes how texting can help users find a wellspring of resilience in moments of crisis in "Spotlight: Texting Through a Crisis."

The Science of Adversity and Resilience

Understanding the biology driving the brain's response to trauma helps identify the right mix of therapies to withstand and recover from adversity. Research over the past two decades has deepened that understanding and provided an evidence base for practice.

Foundational Research

The seminal work of Vincent Felitti, MD, and Robert Anda, MD, on the relationship between adverse childhood experiences (ACEs) and subsequent risk factors for the leading causes of death in adults is well known.[1] Most importantly, Felitti and Anda found that ACEs were common (more than half of adults reported at least one ACE), and that as the number of ACEs increased, so did risky health behaviors and diseases among adults.

In the years since their initial 1998 study, knowledge about how ACEs manifest themselves over time and how the brain is affected by adverse experience has expanded. ACE surveys are now used in many settings throughout the United States and the world.

The groundbreaking work of pediatrician Nadine Burke Harris, MD, MPH, founder of the Center for Youth Wellness in San Francisco, has especially informed research and practice. Burke Harris's focus has been on screening and treatment protocols for children and families living with the effects of toxic stress.[2] As the first California surgeon general (appointed in 2019), Harris has made early childhood, health equity, ACEs, and toxic stress her top policy priorities.[3] Toxic stress results from the overactivation of the body's stress response system, which increases levels of cortisol, adrenaline, and other hormones that can raise heart rate and blood pressure and cause metabolic and immunological effects. Burke Harris has documented that the persistence of such responses can lead to artery-damaging inflammation, which can cause heart disease and stroke; increased risk of learning disabilities, hyperactivity, and anxiety; effects on memory and self-regulation and on physical development; and other long-term conditions.[4] Her research team has identified best measures, practices, and interventions from the now-vast literature on ACEs and their impact on health outcomes, which are available to the field through the National Pediatric Practice Community on Adverse Childhood Experiences.[5]

The Impact of Childhood Maltreatment on the Developing Brain

Neuroscientist Martin Teicher and his colleagues also probe biological response mechanisms, zeroing in on the specific brain changes that occur with different types of maltreatment in childhood. They are especially interested in how a child's susceptibility to psychopathology (i.e., mental health disorders) influences the response.

The specific ways that a child experiences maltreatment will dictate the ways in which the brain changes.[6,7] For example, exposure to high levels of parental verbal abuse alters the language-processing auditory cortex, especially one communication pathway of primary importance. Similarly, children who have witnessed domestic violence exhibit changes in the visual cortex and in the pathway that connects the visual cortex with the limbic system, which is responsible for remembering and responding emotionally to what has been seen. Those who have been sexually abused are affected in the somatosensory cortex, which governs touch and feeling in the genital area.[8]

Maltreatment has very selective effects on the brain.—Martin Teicher

The changes to the sensory systems that result from maltreatment "help the individual cope by turning down how much they're experiencing, at least at the conscious level," Teicher explains. "It makes it easier to get through their childhood."

But in the long term, the effects can be quite damaging. The more the auditory system is turned down, the more verbal comprehension and verbal IQ decline. Likewise, when the visual system is turned down, the part of the brain that is involved in recognizing letters and words is affected, potentially interfering with the ability to read. Somatosensory cortex changes not only may enable a child to endure sexual abuse but also may significantly diminish the ability to experience sexual pleasure in adulthood.

These brain alterations are not likely to be reversed. "The sensory systems seem to have windows in which they're plastic and modifiable by experience and those windows tend to close, generally somewhat after puberty," notes Teicher. "While people can learn to cope and adapt, they can't undo some of the consequences."

The effects of adverse experiences on brain development and the risk for psychopathology are most powerful during sensitive periods, which can vary by gender. For example, abnormalities in the hippocampus, which has a key role in consolidating short-term memory to long-term memory, have been associated with multiple psychiatric conditions. A study looking at childhood neglect and abuse found that the hippocampus in boys was affected by neglect, but not abuse, through age seven.[9] For females, abuse was the significant predictor of hippocampal effect, evident at ages 10 and 11 and again at ages 15 and 16. So there were "completely different stories in males and females," says Teicher.

Maltreatment Alters the Threat Response

"One of the most powerful effects of maltreatment," Teicher says, "is to program how we respond to threat by modifying the amygdala [which has a key role in fear, anxiety, and aggression] and the hypothalamic-pituitary-adrenal axis [which controls reaction to stress and regulates mood and emotion]." Physical maltreatment between ages 3 and 6 and peer emotional abuse (e.g., emotional bullying) at ages 13 and 15 were "the most important predictors of amygdala response."[10]

Prepubertal and postpubertal exposure to maltreatment have opposite effects on amygdala function.[11] The more maltreatment a child experiences when young, the more blunted the amygdala response to threat becomes in adulthood. By contrast, more exposure to emotional bullying in the teen years amplifies the response.

Developmentally these differences are appropriate. If a four-year-old responds too strongly to parents who swing between nurturing and abusive behaviors, the attachment bond might be affected, leaving the child more vulnerable. A teenager, on the other hand, is likely capable of using the fight-or-flight response to deal with bullying, so a stronger reaction makes sense.

But both the blunted and amplified responses to threat pose problems in adulthood. Once grown, an individual with a blunted response may fail to detect danger, increasing the likelihood of engaging in risky activities (e.g., as substance abuse or unprotected sex). And when the response is elevated, a person may misread neutral facial expressions and situations as dangerous, increasing the risk of anxiety or post-traumatic stress disorder.

Maltreatment Changes the Brain, Regardless of Resilience

Teicher and his team expected that the brains of children who had been maltreated but were resilient, demonstrating no clinical signs of psychopathology, would not exhibit the same brain changes as those who did show signs of psychopathology. That hypothesis proved to be wrong.[12] "The global network architecture has changed in maltreated individuals," Teicher reports. "It doesn't matter if you're maltreated and have no symptoms or maltreated and have symptoms."

The most unexpected consequences of our research have to do with the nature of resilience and recovery.—Martin Teicher

In the two maltreated groups, the affected areas of the brain are less fully interconnected, and the nodes that link them do not function normally; conductivity of the neurological signals between the areas is reduced, compared to those who have not been maltreated. But there is still a critical difference. In resilient individuals, the abnormally functioning nodes are even less connected so that the brain changes have less overall impact than they do in susceptible individuals.[13] By studying 14 brain measures, Teicher and his colleagues can predict, with about 80 percent accuracy, not only whether a person was maltreated, but also whether he or she is resilient or susceptible to psychopathology.

Teicher's team also studies what happens to the brains of individuals who recover from maltreatment. These and other insights become the foundation on which to identify the combination of somatic treatments (e.g., pharmaceuticals, neurofeedback), psychotherapies, and social support that is best to bolster resilience.

PACEs: Protecting Against ACEs

While the impact of ACEs is well documented, the influence of positive experiences has been less fully studied. Researchers at Oklahoma State University have taken on the challenge of investigating factors that might mitigate the impact of ACEs and alter a child's trajectory. Amanda Sheffield Morris's research focuses on social and emotional development in children and adolescents and on promoting resilience in high-risk youth and families. Morris and her colleague, Jennifer Hays-Grudo, PhD, developed a model of 10 protective and compensatory experiences (PACEs) that counteract ACEs. The model is built on the importance of "positive relationships and resources that lead to optimal neurodevelopment; social, cognitive, and emotional functioning; healthy behaviors; developmental milestones; and health and longevity," Morris explains.

The most important relationship in a child's life is a caregiver's unconditional love, she says. Indeed, Morris emphasizes, it is "the basis of all development and early attachment." Relationship-based PACEs also include having a best friend, volunteering in the community, having a mentor outside the home, and being active in a social group. Other protective and compensatory factors are resources, such as a safe and clean home, with healthy meals; regular exercise; an engaging hobby; continued opportunities for learning; and regular routines and habits that promote well-being.

The researchers have found that the risk of ACEs can be buffered in vulnerable families by a high level of PACEs.[14] "We know the negative effects of maltreatment but there are healing effects on the brain when you have good relationships and enriching environments," says Morris. While the brain is never fully "healed," it is possible to approach "more normal patterns of networking through positive relationships and directed activities such as those that are built on mindfulness."

Morris thinks of PACEs as "life rafts" that can be extended to children who are adrift in a sea of negative experiences. Viewed as an intervention, the model can point the way to policies that promote the positive relationships, activities, and community involvement that characterize enriched environments.

Parents can view PACEs as a plan for providing an appropriate environment for their children, and the model can offer reassurance as well. People who complete the PACEs survey after the ACEs survey "can see that they're not necessarily doomed," Morris says. One respondent reflected, "I knew about ACEs but once I understood about PACEs it really helped me understand why I am where I am."

The PACEs model is poised for greater attention through multiple new information sources developed by the researchers. A website, *www.acesandpaces.com*, describes the two concepts and provides links to articles, questionnaires, and other resources. A book authored by Hays-Grudo and Morris, *Adverse and Protective Childhood Experiences: A Developmental Perspective*, was published in March 2020,[15] and a new journal, *Adversity and Resilience Science*, launched in April 2020 with articles on protective factors and processes promoting resilience in the face of adversity throughout the life span.[16]

Mitigating Trauma and Fostering Resilience in Girls

As they sharpen their understanding of the biological basis of trauma and recovery, researchers and practitioners are also highlighting the social and cultural contexts in which abuses take place. That framework helps inform mitigation efforts at health clinics, juvenile detention facilities, schools, and elsewhere, where girls are being supported—not punished—for the lives they have led.

Addressing the Impact of Childhood Sexual Abuse

In her role as director of the Mount Sinai Adolescent Health Center in New York, Angela Diaz is particularly familiar with the adolescent experience. The health center provides free, confidential, comprehensive, and integrated services to more than 12,000 young people ages 10 to 26—"head to toes, mental to dental" as Diaz describes it. Almost all (98%) come from low-income families, and 70 percent lack health insurance. They have "very high rates of trauma and social problems that complicate their risks, behaviors, and health needs," explains Diaz. "And they face economic, cultural, racial, and educational barriers that lead to negative lifetime impacts like inter-generational poverty, high pregnancy rates, school dropout, and drug and alcohol abuse." These challenges make it harder for them to flourish and reach the promise of adolescence despite their many strengths.

Despite all of these factors, which can undermine young people's resilience, hope emerges from the Mount Sinai experience. Outcomes are "dramatically improved once these young people find a health home" at the center, Diaz notes. They are more likely than their peers to graduate from high school and attend college and less likely to have an unintended pregnancy.

Every young person wants to be treated in a humane way with dignity. They need to feel that they matter and that people care about them. They need to feel listened to and that they are partners in their care.—Angela Diaz

As part of routine health visits, Diaz and colleagues ask their young patients whether they have ever been sexually abused. Almost one-quarter (23%) of girls say yes, and 66 percent of those report incest. These young people are immediately connected to the center's mental health services, and most of them (81%) take advantage of the counseling available there to address their trauma.

To examine the problem more closely, Diaz obtained detailed data from a sample of 100 girls who had disclosed sexual abuse:

- The mean age at which sexual abuse started was 8.8 years, and for many it was as young as 3, 4, or 5. Many (70%) experienced the first abuse before puberty.
- Two-thirds (67%) reported abuse from one perpetrator, while the others had been abused by multiple perpetrators (an average of three).
- The first perpetrator was most often the biological father (31%), followed by a stepfather or mother's boyfriend (23%). Other family members or individuals known to the family were also frequently the abuser.
- The mean age of the perpetrators was 32. "These are the people who are supposed to love, nurture, and take care of [these children], says Diaz, decrying the imbalance in age, development, and power. "Imagine the impact that has."
- The majority were abused multiple times—monthly, weekly, or even daily. "When do they have the time to go through the normal growth and development young people are supposed to go through?" asks Diaz, more in sadness than true uncertainty.
- In addition to sexual abuse, 68 percent of the girls reported physical abuse, and 59 percent reported emotional abuse.

As Martin Teicher has outlined, the trauma induced by this type, level, and duration of abuse significantly alters brain development. The amygdala of sexually abused young people will be highly activated, generating anxiety and fear. At the same time, the decision-making and regulatory role of the prefrontal cortex will be diminished, leading them to exhibit inappropriate and troubling behavior in school and elsewhere. "We need to understand their behavior in the context of what happened to them and connect them to the services that can be helpful," stressed Diaz.

Diaz compared these 100 girls to 100 other girls who did not report sexual abuse but may have experienced trauma of some kind (70% of youth seen at the health center have a history of some type of trauma). The young women who had been abused were less trusting, communicated less well, felt alienated, and were less connected to their mothers, even if their mothers were not involved in the abuse, compared to those who had not been sexually abused. Many had run away from home. The abused girls also had a lower sense of self and were more likely to be depressed. Some 85 percent had thought of suicide, and 42 percent had attempted suicide anywhere from one to seven times, with pills being the most common method used.

These findings were consistent with a study conducted by Diaz and colleagues using a nationally representative sample of 3,015 girls in grades five through 12.[17] Ten percent of them disclosed a history of childhood sexual abuse. They had poorer mental health and were more likely to smoke, drink, use drugs, or engage in food binging or purging, compared with those reporting no abuse. The impact was much greater for the 5 percent who had also been physically abused. Yet only 27 percent of the abused girls had seen a mental health counselor for any reason.

Young people who have been sexually abused may never have disclosed the abuse to others or may not have been believed by family or other adults to whom they did confide. Asking about abuse in an empathic, nonjudgmental way in the context of a health visit, says Diaz, provides "an opportunity for young people to disclose and for the health care provider or mental health clinician to let them know that this has happened to many other children and youth, it is not something they did wrong, and it is the responsibility of the person who abused them."

Regarding the long-term effects of trauma, Diaz notes that "life is a one-way street and there is no such thing as true reversal. Rather, resilience and recovery can help change a child's trajectory for the positive." She stresses the value of patient-centered integrated services, such as those provided at Mount Sinai Adolescent Health Center.

Understanding How Girls Experience Trauma, Racism, and Resilience

Applauding Diaz's work, attorney Rebecca Epstein, the executive director of the Center on Poverty and Inequality at Georgetown Law, observed that research, in general, tends to focus on boys or to be gender neutral. "Girls' experiences are unique," she says, yet they are understudied.

> When considering resilience, girls in particular, especially girls of color, low-income girls, and rural girls have remained invisible and pushed to the margins of the conversation.—Rebecca Epstein

Trauma and its influence on girls' involvement with the juvenile justice system and with school discipline is a particular concern to Epstein. She noted a study by the National Institute of Justice that illustrated the association between the experience of ACEs and contact with the juvenile justice system: Youth who had been abused and neglected were 59 percent more likely to be arrested as a juvenile.[18]

But the occurrence of ACEs among girls was found to be stunningly higher than among boys. A study of 64,329 youth in the Florida juvenile justice system showed that[19]:

- Almost half (46%) of girls had five or more ACEs, compared to 28 percent of boys.
- Girls were more likely than boys to have had each of the 10 categories of ACEs.
- The starkest difference was in the experience of sexual abuse: 31 percent of girls reported being sexually abused compared with 7 percent of boys.

"Damaging though they can be, household-based ACEs are not the exclusive source of trauma," warns Epstein. A wider societal context brings other potentially scarring experiences to the fore. The traditional ACE categories, for example, do not capture the experience of girls "who survive sexual violence outside of the home, gender inequities throughout our public systems and workplaces, and the societal factors that come into play when you identify as a girl," says Epstein. Nor do they encompass the "historical and cultural trauma of racism that is sewn into our culture for girls of color who carry the legacy of hundreds of years of racism including, for many, being treated as hypersexualized and as fundamentally less human." Emerging ACEs scales are expanding the scope beyond the household environment to include community, institutional, and systemic factors, such as exposure to community violence and school bullying.[20]

Racism against Black girls, in particular, is rooted in stereotypes of Black women that are omnipresent—including the architypes of the angry Black woman, the strong Black woman, and the sexualized Black woman—and tend to be projected onto Black girls. This leads to "adultification bias" in which people in positions of authority view Black girls and young women as less innocent than White girls of the same age.[21]

> *Black girls are often not viewed as fundamentally human and not afforded the leniency given to White girls. Black girls' tears are not valued the way we value White girls' tears because we associate White girls with an innocence that engenders compassion and sympathy by adults.*—Rebecca Epstein

By dehumanizing Black girls and holding them to adult-like standards of behavior, adultification bias contributes to harsher punishment by institutions and authority figures.

Criminalizing Sexually Abused Girls

The experience of sexual abuse is deeply rooted in our history and culture, and for Black girls it is also linked to "the legacy of slavery and the commodification of Black women's and girls' bodies," Epstein stresses.

Sexual abuse leads girls into a "truly egregious cycle," says Epstein, describing a "sexual abuse to prison pipeline" in which "girls are criminalized for the sexual abuse that they experience and assigned complicity in their victimization." All too often, their reports of sexual abuse are not believed, and girls of color are not recognized as crime survivors but are instead blamed for the violence they have endured.

The most glaring example is victims of sex trafficking, the vast majority of whom are girls of color. They are often arrested for prostitution and related charges and brought into the juvenile justice system when "they are, in fact, survivors of rape for profit," states Epstein unequivocally. Typically, the pimps and the buyers who treat girls as a marketable commodity are not held accountable.

Once in the system, girls are often exposed to conditions that trigger or worsen past trauma symptoms. With few opportunities for the counseling, connection, education, and skills building that might help a young woman begin to heal, they may instead engage in behaviors on release that return them to detention, entering what Epstein describes as "a negative, downward spiral that began as a traumatic experience that needed to be healed and supported rather than punished."

Criminalizing Status and School-Related Offenses

Girls are also disproportionately punished for age-related status offenses, such as truancy, drinking, or curfew violations. A girl might escape an abusive home and then be remanded to juvenile justice as a runaway rather than receive help. When that happens, "She is being routed into the system for escaping violence," laments Epstein.

> It's not the behavior that's the problem; it's our response. And the risk is that we're not seeing these girls for who they are and what has happened to them.
> —Rebecca Epstein

School disciplinary codes address transgressions that are often subjectively determined, such as disrupting school, showing disrespect, or not adhering to a dress code. These violations are vulnerable to bias in how they are interpreted, and indeed, research indicates that Black girls are judged to be violating these codes more often than White girls.[22] Stationing police officers at a school also drives girls into the justice system because their involvement facilitates entry into juvenile detention rather than the principal's office.

Helping Girls Build Resilience

A first step toward overcoming these harmful responses to girls of color, and one that many well-intentioned people miss, is to "bring girls' voices to the forefront and recognize that we need to listen before we can support," Epstein says. (The theme of directly engaging the populations most affected by challenges under discussion echoes throughout this volume. See, for example, chapter 4: "Immigrants in America: Stories of Trauma and Resilience," and chapter 8: "Home, the Heart of Place").

The right training for teachers, school administrators, police officers, and others "who wield such influence over the trajectories of girls' lives," is also key, she adds. With guidance, they can become "more culturally competent, trauma-informed, and gender-responsive, so they are looking through a cross-section of lenses that include sex, gender identity, race, ethnicity, sexual orientation, and trauma." Epstein believes that is "the most upstream method for preventing the cycle of trauma being criminalized."

Better data collection is a further step. Schools and the federal government are not collecting data that are disaggregated by race, gender, and offense, information that is needed to isolate bias and harmful disciplinary patterns. "If we don't center research questions on girls," said Epstein, "their lot is not going to improve." And where discriminatory patterns emerge, action needs to be taken.

Resilience Within the Juvenile Justice System

About half the states allow status offenders to be put into the juvenile justice system, even though these offenses rarely involve a threat to public safety. Closing what Epstein and other advocates call a "status offense loophole" is essential to reduce contact with criminal justice, especially for girls of color.

Sending young girls into the system for prostitution, meanwhile, ignores their vulnerability as children who do not even have a legally recognized capacity to consent to sex. Rethinking responses to sex trafficking and focusing more on the demand for paid sex and the people who are selling the girls are important ways to reduce the trauma of further rape and accompanying abuse.

Circling back to the biology of abuse, Epstein believes policies that will support girls and enable them to thrive start "with a recognition of trauma and adversity and how they affect the brain and behavior, using that as a basis to create approaches to girls in developmentally appropriate and trauma-informed ways" so that they can begin to tap into their own resilient strength.

Resilience Within the Schools

School policies and practices can assist girls further upstream and better connect them to their school community and buttress academic success, rather than isolating them. Mental health counseling and cognitive behavioral therapy are important modules to help girls succeed. And gender-responsive mind/body programs, such as mindfulness, meditation, and yoga, can provide safe spaces that promote self-regulation and healing.

The in-school police presence that militarizes the school environment does not help establish trusting relationships and truly safe spaces for students. In conversations across the country, Epstein and colleagues have heard girls say that police do not make their lives safer, but instead impede their ability to be themselves, free of surveillance. Police may interact with girls in ways that "reinforce stereotypes based on traditional White cultural norms of femininity," says Epstein. The recent uprisings in the aftermath of the police killing of George Floyd have increased awareness of disproportionate police violence against communities of color and responsive policies, but girls of color are not often part of the conversation.

A further obstacle to resilient development is that teachers and other school staff may be dealing with their own trauma or with secondary trauma rooted in their interactions with students. Without opportunities for healing and self-care, their ability to provide the compassion, patience, and generosity required to interact with traumatized students may be significantly compromised.

Epstein recommends restorative justice as a "transformative tool" that engages students and teachers in resolving harm, creating community, and building relationships.[23] Done well, restorative justice, with its focus on repairing and rebuilding rather than destroying or punishing, creates a supportive environment in which peers and teachers listen, respond, and connect. Students are more likely to thrive in such a climate and feel more connected to their schools. "School connectedness is a key determinant of academic success, and education is a key social determinant of health," Epstein notes.

Many interventions targeting young people who have experienced trauma have been deficit based, focusing on what is "wrong" or "missing" about youth and their lives. Epstein advocates for a different approach, one that recognizes and cultivates the strength and resilience that girls already possess, helping to create the sense of agency and empowerment that is key to fostering resilience.

Above all, we need to listen to youth when we're crafting policies and program-matic solutions.—Rebecca Epstein

A Final Word

Girls experience adversity and trauma in ways and degrees that are different from the experience of boys. Giving voice to their experiences and understanding the underlying basis for their reaction to trauma will help reduce the negative impact of these experiences and open up pathways to resilience.

Ongoing research is yielding an ever-deeper and more nuanced understanding of the complicated short- and long-term effects of adverse experiences on the architecture of the developing brain. Exciting new developments are illuminating the biological underpinnings of resilience, with the hope of identifying targeted approaches to help individuals recover from their trauma.

Armed with this knowledge, those who care for girls can better help them understand past adversity and point the way toward a more successful future. For girls of color in particular, the need is especially urgent so they are not lost in the aftermath of trauma. With compassionate attention that recognizes their humanity and listens and responds to their voices, girls can uncover and strengthen their own resilience. The science provides the evidence.

Spotlight

Texting Through a Crisis

Bob Filbin, MA, Chief Data Scientist and Co-Founder, Crisis Text Line

In the darkest moments of their lives, young people are finding help through the Crisis Text Line ("text HOME to 741741").[1] Now available in the United States, Canada, Ireland, and the United Kingdom, the resource provides access to trained crisis counselors who respond to texters around the clock, helping them to move beyond a crisis. Most people learn about the Crisis Text Line through social media.

In contrast to telephone-based helplines, a person can send a confidential text from anywhere—the school cafeteria, a bedroom, even the bathroom. Because young people trust texting, they may be willing to use the service where they might be reluctant to turn to more traditional services.

In its seven years of operation, Crisis Text Line crisis counselors have exchanged more than 160 million messages globally. According to Crisis Text Line's survey data (about 21% of texters submit the survey), 75 percent of texters are under the age of 25, and 15 percent are 13 and under. Many texters in the youngest group (13 and under) are at high risk, with 20 percent indicating that they are engaged in cutting themselves or other self-harm. Often underserved, Native American and Latino texters account for 25 percent of total users. About 28 percent of U.S. texters report living in households with less than $20,000 annual income.

Trained Crisis Counselors Provide Critical Connection

More than 35,000 volunteers have completed Crisis Text Line's 35-hour online training program. Since both training and counseling can be done from anywhere an internet connection is available, "We have volunteers who are bedridden, active military, or live in extremely rural areas—people who wouldn't otherwise be able to volunteer for a crisis center," says Filbin.

Bob Filbin, *Spotlight: Texting Through a Crisis* In: *Community Resilience.* Edited by: Alonzo L. Plough, Oxford University Press (2021). © Robert Wood Johnson Foundation. DOI: 10.1093/oso/9780197559383.003.0009

Crisis counselors must be at least 18 years old and undergo a background check. Assessment standards are strict, and only about a third of applicants become crisis counselors. Once approved, crisis counselors commit to four hours weekly and stay between six and eight months on average. As of June 2020, about 10,000 crisis counselors were active each month across the countries served.

Two core skills keep the focus on the texter: active listening (fully concentrating on what the texter is saying, rather than thinking about what to say next) and collaborative problem-solving (letting the texter take the lead on solution ideas as a pathway to empowerment). Common across people in crisis is a desire for connection, observes Filbin; in fact, 68 percent of texter survey respondents say they shared feelings they have never shared with another person before.

People in crisis want not only specific skills. They also want to connect with somebody. Human connection is at the center of Crisis Text Line's work.—Bob Filbin

Collecting Data in Real Time

To assess outcomes, Crisis Text Line asks texters to complete a survey at the end of the exchange that uses validated indicators to measure reductions in crisis and suicide risk. The data, says Filbin, show "that 86 percent of respondents see an improvement in their scores on these measures—a proxy of our ability to move people out of crisis."

Rather than look back at a moment of crisis, as traditional surveys do, Crisis Text Line data "provide a unique perspective on crisis in three ways: they include real-time data, the words of the user, in the moment of crisis," Filbin emphasizes. "Those three attributes make our data a useful complement to surveys, with the goal of preventing and intervening in crises."

Using the 140 million-message database (in the United States), which maintains strict data security and texter privacy, Crisis Text Line's data science team conducts its own internal research and uses a triage tool to identify texters at high risk for suicide attempts, moving them to the head of the queue. The data also allow the project to pinpoint moments of highest need and adjust staffing appropriately. (For more on issues surrounding the ever-expanding use of digital data, see chapter 13: "Digital Data, Ethical Challenges.")

External researchers are critical partners in special projects. "We use the research to not only improve our service but to share insights with the crisis space as a whole," stresses Filbin. For example, the Crisis Text Line is working with the Veterans Administration to develop an algorithm that identifies suicide risk in veterans.

As of June 2020, Crisis Text Line had 12 published research papers and expected another six to be published before the end of the year. Topics include:

- *Text patterns in youth following the suicides of Anthony Bourdain and Kate Spade and the release of 13 Reasons Why, a television series about teen suicide. (Crisis Text Line was featured as a resource in season two of 13 Reasons Why.)[2,3]*
- *The association between temperature in the United States and the extent to which young adults and adolescents seek crisis support.[4]*
- *Geographic trends across the rural-urban continuum in the use of Crisis Text Line.[5]*
- *Crisis Text Line is growing rapidly, with plans to expand to provide global coverage in Spanish, French, Portuguese, and Standard Arabic within the next five years. At the same time the service seeks to become more deeply integrated into communities.*

We want to be where people in crisis are: in every school bathroom, at every bus stop, every place where somebody could need crisis support—a service that's always at people's fingertips.—Bob Filbin

Home, the Heart of Place

Lisa Dubay, PhD, Senior Fellow, Urban Institute and Co-director, National Coordinating Center for Policies for Action

Andre Perry, PhD, David M. Rubenstein Fellow, Metropolitan Policy Program, the Brookings Institution

Assata Richards, PhD, Director of the Sankofa Research Institute

Brian Smedley, PhD, Chief of psychology in the public interest, American Psychological Association

"Our homes are more than sticks and nails," declares Carlos Martin, PhD, a senior fellow at the Urban Institute and a trained architect. In framing housing as a pillar of well-being, he adds, "Homes are places for reflection, family, and community. Homes are financial and cultural assets. Homes are platforms for other life outcomes, like health, education, and jobs."

Or, as Dorothy remarked more plaintively in *The Wizard of Oz*, "There is no place like home."

But home is also a place that for many reflects a confluence of systemic injustices, government policy, and private-sector development decisions steeped in structural racism. The housing situation for many people of color across America today tells, in part, a story about inequities that have never been fully acknowledged and persistent discriminatory practices. Soaring housing prices and enduring income and educational disparities further fuel the inability of vast numbers of people to find housing they can afford and in neighborhoods that don't face structural disadvantages.

During a conversation at the 2019 *Sharing Knowledge* conference about the imperative of stable housing, an audience member offered a deeply personal description of the home her family had lost. It had been destroyed as part of a government-sanctioned urban renewal process of the 1960s, which razed center-city neighborhoods across the country:

Lisa Dubay, Andre Perry, Assata Richards, and Brian Smedley, *Home, the Heart of Place* In: *Community Resilience.* Edited by: Alonzo L. Plough, Oxford University Press (2021). © Robert Wood Johnson Foundation. DOI: 10.1093/oso/9780197559383.003.0010

The home that I grew up in was taken by urban renewal, six months after my parents had "burned the mortgage," as they called it. My mother never recovered from that. And it killed her. She literally mourned herself to death because at the age they should have been getting ready and preparing for retirement in their little castle, here comes this thing called urban renewal.

Took our home, destroyed our neighborhood—and it has impacted my life, all the days of my life ever since. So, yes, it is trauma. And that trauma is driven through policies. And it begins at the planning table.

This poignant saga sets the stage for understanding the mix of emotional ties and survival benefits that accrue from healthy and affordable housing—and the consequences when it is missing.

Brian Smedley, presenting in his capacity as executive director of the National Collaborative for Health Equity (he has since changed positions), opens the chapter with a look at the nation's shameful record of discrimination and disinvestment, which has concentrated poverty in so many communities of color today. Next, the Urban Institute's Lisa Dubay highlights the many strands of research at the intersection of health and housing. Assata Richards of the Sankofa Research Institute and Andre Perry of the Brookings Institution both celebrate the resilience of communities of color and the often-unrecognized assets embedded there. Richards speaks to the cultural history that so enriches a neighborhood and lifts up the ethical imperative of conducting research in ways that benefit the people being studied, while Perry looks at how Black communities have been devalued in the marketplace and explains what it takes for residents to demand their fair price.

The Housing Challenge Today

Viewed from almost any angle, this nation has a housing crisis. Certainly, it is evident from the vantage point of affordability. Half of all renter households in the United States, and one-third of owner households, spend more than 30 percent of their income on housing, a figure that approaches 70 percent among low-income households.[1]

Understanding the intertwined threads that have fostered the housing patterns we see today encourages "us to be rabble rousers," proclaims Brian Smedley. In particular, the increasing concentration of poverty over the past 40 years emerges as prominent and troubling. From 1970 to 2010, the number of households living in both medium-poverty census tracts (defined as those in which between 20 and 30 percent of residents are below the poverty line) and high-poverty tracts (where 30 percent or more of the population is poor) has risen steadily. And in the first decade of the 21st century, neighborhoods in extreme poverty (40% of the population living below poverty) also increased, a trend likely to have worsened since the housing crash a decade ago.[2]

People of color disproportionately dwell in these communities. About 40 percent of Black households in metropolitan areas are in census tracts with medium or high rates of poverty, compared to about 10 percent of White households. A look only at families below the poverty line reveals a similar trend. About 70 percent of low-income White families live in low-poverty census tracts (where the concentration of poverty is below 20 percent), while only one-third of similarly poor Blacks do so.[3]

While differences in income, education, and wealth among these populations undoubtedly contribute to that concentration, it also reflects persisting patterns of segregation. These data, says Smedley, reflect "our history of sorting people into different neighborhoods, sometimes by law and practices, sometimes by custom, and sometimes even after our fair-housing laws outlawed it, through discriminatory practices in real estate, home lending, and rental properties."

Deliberate and long-standing economic disinvestment in communities of color fostered the residential patterns in place now. Redlining, for example, goes back to the 1930s, when the federal government and private banks flagged certain neighborhoods as "high risk," denying them access to mortgages and discouraging investment. We also live with the legacies of racist zoning practices, the concentration of public housing in already-impoverished neighborhoods, and the subsidies that were allocated to builders to develop Whites-only suburbs. The damage wrought by restrictive covenants, tax exemptions, and loan patterns that enforced segregation, and by the violence that emerged in response to integration, have not been repaired.

> *When we see that kind of systematic disadvantage against a neighborhood, we need to understand that these patterns occurred within the lifetimes of people living today and the consequences carry forward.*—Brian Smedley

The wealth gap remains a particularly clear-cut result of long-standing inequities in housing policy. Because Black people were barred from purchasing homes in many desirable neighborhoods, they were never able to benefit from increasing property values or pass along a significant asset to their children. "It's one of the biggest explanations for the wealth gap between White and Black and White and Brown families that we see today," Smedley points out. That, too, was intensified by the housing crash of 2008.

Highlights From the Research

The health consequences that flow from this mix of forces can be all too easily captured in one compelling data point: Overlay a map of the racial composition in Baltimore with another showing life expectancy and what emerges is a nearly 30-year longevity difference across certain census tracts, with residents of highly segregated Black neighborhoods invariably experiencing shorter life spans.[4]

As a framework for thinking about the many intersections of health and housing at the neighborhood level, Smedley presented a structural analysis by George Galster, PhD, an urban policy expert at Wayne State University in Detroit. Galster identified four mechanisms through which neighborhoods influence health and well-being, as well as economic and educational opportunities[5]:

- **Social interactive mechanisms** include the norms, attitudes, and behaviors that dictate what is acceptable and the social cohesion that enables neighbors to come together to solve collective challenges.
- **Environmental mechanisms**, such as pollution, toxic exposure, blight, violence, and adverse childhood experiences, can stoke distrust, stress, and social isolation.
- **Geographical forces** can drive investment decisions, such as encouraging polluting industries and others that contribute to environmental degradation to site their operations in neighborhoods likely to lack the political power to resist them.
- And finally, **institutional mechanisms**, from stigmatizing a community and its residents to resource-poor educational systems and inequitable criminal and juvenile justice policies, can discourage investment.

The multidimensional interactions among these forces suggest the need for deeper research across the health and housing fields. Structural deficits, leading to the presence of pests and mold and chipping lead paint, are particularly obvious points of overlap. The rent burdens that make it difficult for individuals or families to afford health-related expenses also suggest interconnected challenges, as do the stress and depression associated with housing instability. In communities that are starved of the infrastructure and public safety investments that help stabilize housing, other health issues inevitably surface.

And, with homelessness increasingly visible in countless cities, the health consequences of having no shelter at all are painfully apparent. Chicago is just one example: Researchers reported that nearly half the individuals who make frequent visits to the University of Illinois/Chicago hospital emergency room are homeless.[6]

Policies for Action: Key Findings

Under the umbrella of the *Policies for Action* initiative funded by the Robert Wood Johnson Foundation (RWJF), research collaborators are already examining the interwoven nature of health and housing. In particular, they are looking at how health is influenced by federally subsidized housing, low-income housing tax credits, and initiatives to renovate deteriorating public housing. Scholars are also examining the impact of gentrification on the health of low-income children and taking a qualitative look at initiatives that bring the two sectors together. Lisa Dubay, who co-directs the national coordinating center for *Policies for Action*, summarizes some of that research:

- **Among children, living in federally subsidized housing is associated with missing fewer days of school, a lower chance of being unhappy or depressed, and a greater likelihood of being well behaved.** Urban Institute researchers reached those conclusions using a unique data set that linked the National Health Interview Survey (a broad range of health information collected in household interviews) to Housing and Urban Development (HUD) statistics.
- **Adults who receive more housing assistance are less likely to delay health care due to cost and face less food insecurity, compared to adults who receive less such assistance.** This suggests people may be using the savings that accrue from rental subsidies to pay for other basic needs. Those findings, drawn from the linked data set described previously, are based on an analysis by researchers at the Boston University School of Social Work.[7]
- **There aren't enough housing vouchers to go around, and even when vouchers are available, the housing for which individuals and families are eligible might not be.** While federally subsidized housing vouchers are a key mechanism for securing affordable housing, they are in limited supply. In contrast to Medicare and Medicaid, which are entitlement programs available to anyone who meets their eligibility criteria, only about one-quarter of the population receives the federal vouchers for which they qualify.[8]

  Moreover, housing is hard to secure even with those vouchers.[9] Researchers looked at initiatives in Vancouver, Wash., which prioritizes medically complex individuals and homeless families with school-age children for vouchers, and in Portland, Ore., which targets seniors and people with disabilities. Analysis of the health impacts among those populations is ongoing, but the study has already concluded that only 30 percent of those eligible in Vancouver and 25 percent of those in Portland were actually able to obtain housing.[10]

- **Some states are using health-promoting criteria to assess and award federal low-income housing tax credits to developers.**[11] Scholars at the University of Florida and the University of Illinois found that more than half the states are going well beyond standard building codes in determining eligibility for tax credits, using the tools of green building certification, standard setting, and "qualified allocation plans" that specify award priorities. Many require building materials and practices that minimize moisture, mold, allergens, and toxicity; mandate appropriate indoor air flow and ventilation; and emphasize resident safety.

- **Renovating public housing offers health benefits.** Across the country, the need to renovate public housing is vast and unmet: The New York City Housing Authority alone estimates that it will need $31.8 billion over five years to restore the infrastructure of some 2,400 buildings.[12] Using Medicaid claims data, researchers at the New York University Wagner School of Public Policy followed residents in six public housing apartment buildings before and after they were renovated. While they did not find changes in specific housing-sensitive conditions (asthma, anxiety or depression, upper respiratory infection, or injury), they did document improvements in an overall index that combined these conditions.[13]

- **Upper respiratory infections, asthma, mood disorders, and chronic respiratory diseases are "persistently and uniquely" associated with substandard housing in low-income populations.**[14] Researchers used machine-learning resources to link the claims of more than one million Medicaid enrollees living in New York City from 2006 to 2017 with data from the U.S. Census Bureau's American Community Survey (a key source of population and housing information) and from housing violations and building complaints. The preliminary conclusions may give cities new incentive for identifying housing that is in need of repair or renovation.

- **"The relationship between neighborhood economic change and health may be more nuanced than is often assumed."**[15] That conclusion, published in a *Health Affairs* analysis, reflected an analysis of the impact of gentrification on children, drawing from Medicaid data. In 82 rapidly gentrifying census tracts in New York State, there were relatively small differences in measures of overweight or obesity, asthma, hospitalization, or emergency department use by children ages 9 to 11. There were, however, increases in the rates at which they were diagnosed with anxiety and depression.

Another piece of research, presented at one of the 2019 *Sharing Knowledge* poster sessions, underscores the power of political will in addressing some of the nation's most pressing housing challenges. In Los Angeles, a public/private package of investments funded supportive housing for more than 3,000 homeless individuals with complex health and social service needs. A year after being housed through this flexible funding pool, a RAND evaluation found that emergency room visits had fallen by 67.5 percent, hospital inpatient days by 76.5 percent, and the need for mental health crisis stabilization by 59.5 percent.[16]

The Power of Community Ties

From that broad-based overview of key research, Assata Richards took an in-depth look at the Third Ward, one of Houston's oldest African-American communities. The childhood home of musicians from Lightnin' Hopkins to Beyoncé, the Third Ward has 4,000 residents, three-quarters of them Black, and is spread across an area of about half of a square mile. By many metrics, not only is it a profoundly economically disadvantaged neighborhood, but also it is also a place where generations of families have forged deep ties. In recent years, the Third Ward has faced what Richards calls "an appetite for gentrification."

Reflecting on housing as "more than just a place to stay," Richards argues that a neighborhood cannot be measured merely by school ratings or crime statistics. She offers insights gleaned not only from an academic career and a prior role as vice chair of the Houston Housing Authority, but also from the personal experience of living in the Third Ward as a third-generation resident.

"What does housing mean in the context of an historical and culturally rich community?" she asks, before suggesting the answer. "It is a connection and an opportunity to be part of a neighborhood that has social capital, where you are supporting one another and being cared for by one another."

Healthy housing is housing that allows you to stay connected to a place that has deep meaning and value for you, where there is a strong sense of collective responsibility for one another.—Assata Richards

Value is measured not only by realtors, but also by residents; not only by what the market will pay, but also by what its inhabitants contribute. The bottom line, says Richards, looks very different "when we see a community through the eyes of its residents, as opposed to the eyes of the real estate market."

Gathering Knowledge to Inform Social Action

With gentrification pressures pushing against the Third Ward, the Sankofa Research Institute, which Richards directs, forged a memorandum of understanding with the Emancipation Economic Development Council, a collaborative dedicated to preserving and revitalizing the Third Ward. Together, they embarked on a research collaboration with Quianta Moore at Rice University's Baker Institute.

Intrinsic to the work, which began in 2018, was respect and empathy for the people of the Third Ward. "When we want to work with our community, we need to let them set the agenda," she says. The first questions to ask residents are, "What do you want? What do you need?" (See chapter 1: "The Storytellers," especially the work of Walter Flores in Guatemala and Julie Rusk in Santa Monica, for related insights about community engagement, the cornerstone of fostering equitable and inclusive.)

To tease out some of the answers, local residents were recruited, trained, and paid a living wage to conduct a door-to-door survey, and the neighbors who spoke with them were paid $50 for their participation. "As a rule, I don't collect data, I don't utilize people's knowledge and information, without compensating them, in the same way we don't do work as researchers unless we are compensated," Richards insists.

Leveling the playing field between study subjects and researchers makes it easier to talk candidly, and Richards emphasizes the message it sends: "We honor you, we respect you, we have empathy with your experience and your dignity and the story you are going to tell us."

> *Collective efficacy takes relationships, sharing the neighborhood, going to school together, being together in a place. That is what history and culture do, it unites us.*—Assata Richards

Equally important is a solutions-oriented approach that empowers residents to preserve, protect, and revitalize their own neighborhood. "The research has to come in conjunction with work around social change and impact," Richards believes fervently. "To go in only to fulfill our curiosity or to obtain knowledge that won't lead to direct action is ethically irresponsible. It builds people's hope if you come out and ask them what they need." (See chapter 13: "Digital Data, Ethical Challenges," which explores the framework for considering this kind of issue.)

> *For us, it's always connecting the work to a social action, not in the end, but in the beginning. I really push back on scholars and individuals coming to study the problem without a clear conceptualization of any solution.*—Assata Richards

Poverty, Passion, and the Power of Community

The Sankofa/Rice University survey garnered responses from more than 1,600 heads of households in the Third Ward.[17] Almost half (47%) of the residents had annual household incomes below $10,000, and an additional 16.3 percent earned between $10,000 and $20,000. Only 26 percent had full-time work, 18 percent were unable to work because of a health-related issue, and about half had experienced food insecurity. Eighty percent were renters, almost one-quarter of whom had seen their monthly rent increase over the past year, and that same percentage worried about having to move in the next 12 months. All of those are concrete indicators of a population highly vulnerable to housing upheaval.

More than 80 percent of residents said they would walk or bike in their neighborhood more often if the infrastructure was improved; 35 percent reported being limited by a fear of crime. Those kinds of findings shift the locus of concern away from the individual and onto the settings they inhabit. "Often times we think we have to bring information to communities," observes Richards. What became apparent in a more careful conversation are the structural barriers to pursuing health. The message surveyors heard from residents is, "You don't even have to tell us we should walk. We want to. Just fix the streets. Fix the sidewalks. Let us walk more."

Housing quality is another key health concern. Alarmingly, 43 percent of residents report pests, 23 percent have mold in their homes, and a significant percentage lack basic amenities—10 percent have no heat or air conditioning, and 7 percent do not have running water.

Despite severe resource limitations, 69 percent of residents do have health insurance, although only 52 percent have a primary care provider, and 8.5 percent say they could not see a mental health professional as needed. The many challenges in their lives perhaps make it somewhat surprising that 54 percent indicate that they are in good or very good health, although diabetes, hypertension, obesity, asthma, and heart conditions are significant contributors to morbidity, roughly in sync with national indicators.

Against all of that emerges a data point that Richards calls a "shining jewel": 80 percent of residents in the Third Ward are satisfied with living in the neighborhood. "You can't buy that number," she marvels. "The value of the neighborhood is beyond all of the demographics and the challenges."

Civic engagement is particularly vigorous, as indicated by the finding that 69 percent of residents voted in the 2016 presidential election, and by social capital, which measures how people feel about the trust and interdependence in their neighborhood. Eighty-seven percent said they believed that local residents would check on an elderly neighbor, 82 percent believed someone would watch a neighbor's child, and most believed that people in their community were willing to give a neighbor a ride or check someone's mail.

What that tells us, says Richards, is that the resilient people who inhabit the Third Ward can make it a better place to live, and that they must be allowed to stay there as it grows more attractive to outsiders. "We have to invest in afford-able housing in neighborhoods that are challenged by gentrification and have a strong legacy of history and culture. We're not just investing in a unit, we're investing in the building blocks of a great neighborhood," she says.

> We came to these places against all odds, in times that people didn't want us. We stayed there when everyone left us there. And we made something beautiful of these places. It is a social justice issue.—Assata Richards

For that reason, Richards has strong reservations about Moving to Opportunity, an ambitious federal initiative designed to help low-income families with chil-dren leave high-poverty neighborhoods. Research to measure the effects of Moving to Opportunity uncovered a package of mixed results. Families who had moved to lower poverty neighborhoods had less obesity, depression, and mental distress and higher incomes. Children benefitted by attending college at higher rates if they moved before reaching age 13, and they were less likely to become single parents as adults. At the same time, the data pointed to negative long-term impacts, especially among children older than 13, possibly because of the dis-ruptive effects of a move.[18]

Through her lens, Richards sees those findings as a clear indication that housing mobility is not a panacea. "The model says that place is the only im-portant thing—schools, transportation, maybe job opportunities," worries Richards. She fears that "the history and culture and the social structure of the community, the social capital" are being left out of the equation.

Rather than encouraging people to leave their community ties behind, Richards favors a formula that includes sharing actionable data, expanding ties to civic groups, building leadership skills, alerting local people when affordable housing comes online, and supporting community self-determination at every turn. What else does it take? Assata's answer: "Patience, a sense of empathy, and a willingness to be flexible to really build authentic, power-sharing, equitable relationships where you are creating together."

Owning a Home While Black

Like Richards, Brookings Institution researcher Andre Perry honors the assets embedded in Black communities. The wellspring of his work is the recognition that those assets tend to be overlooked in policy conversations, and that false assumptions about deficits limit the opportunities available to those who live there. "From a methodological standpoint, we start with the premise that Black people are not broken, Black homes are not broken, Black decisions are not cat-egorically wrong," he says.

We assume that assets in the Black community are strong, that there is nothing wrong with the Black community that ending racism can't solve.—Andre Perry

Persuasive data confirm that the price of housing in a neighborhood goes down as the percentage of Black people living in it rises.[19] In an analysis drawn from the American Community Survey, Perry found that median home values are about $307,000 in areas where the Black population is less than 1 percent. By striking contrast, where Black residents comprise half the population or more, the average value is just under $150,000.

The pat explanation is that communities dominated by Blacks have more crime, poorer schools, and fewer amenities. But after controlling for those factors, a fuller explanation comes into view: "Homes in Black neighborhoods are worth 23 percent less, on average, simply because of the percent of Black folks around them," states Perry. "Not because of the housing structure, not because of the education, not because of crime, but simply because there are Black people in them."

That represents a cumulative total of $156 billion in lost value, a figure that Perry says could pay the price of 8.1 million four-year college degrees or the purchase of 4.4 million Black-owned businesses; replace the water pipes in Flint, Michigan, 3,000 times over; or repair virtually all of the damage wrought by Hurricane Katrina in the Gulf region. "You could buy or start a business, send your kids to college, move out of the neighborhood, improve your home, buy into health care plans," says Perry. "Homes are such a central part of our social structure because the equity essentially funds social services. They enable people to uplift themselves."

The monies that are pulled or robbed from communities because of racism are the things that would improve the social determinants that predict health.—Andre Perry

Like Smedley, Perry calls out racism past and present to explain this devaluation of Black people and the places they live. While the federal Fair Housing Act outlaws explicit discrimination, home buying remains a highly subjective process that readily accommodates other forms of bias. "Real estate agents still steer Black folks in one direction, White folks in another," says Perry. Recapping the many assumptions and behaviors that distort property values, he adds, "We just came off a housing crisis predicated on distributing bad loans to, in general, Black and Brown people. The appraisal process is fraught with all kinds of racial bias."

That creates a new age of redlining. You don't necessarily have to draw the red line on the maps, but guess what: it's very easy to re-create them in other ways.—Andre Perry

Indeed, a powerful, three-year investigation by *Newsday*, published in November 2019, offered clear indication that flagrant violations of the Fair Housing Act continue to this day.[20] The study was conducted on Long Island, a New York City suburb that is one of the most segregated in the United States. Using a "dissimilarity index," the newspaper first sent White homebuyers to real estate agents, and then sent Black, Hispanic, or Asian homebuyers to those same agents. Potential buyers who are Black were treated differently from Whites about half the time (Hispanics were treated differently 39% of the time, and Asians 19%). Disparate treatments included steering people of color to different neighborhoods, offering them fewer listings, and asking that they meet additional financial criteria.

"In one of the most concentrated investigations of discrimination by real estate agents in the half century since enactment of America's landmark fair housing law," declares the newspaper, "*Newsday* found evidence of widespread separate and unequal treatment of minority potential homebuyers and minority communities on Long Island." While not published in a peer-reviewed journal, *Newsday* reported in detail on its methodology, which incorporated a "paired-testing" method that has been recognized by the courts as the only viable way to detect violations of fair housing laws. The newspaper's analysis attracted broad media coverage and led to state Senate hearings.

Against this backdrop of discrimination in so many forms, Perry details a new paradigm for maximizing equity in Black communities in his book, *Know Your Price: Valuing Black Lives and Property in America's Black Cities.*[21] Factoring in core assets that are generally left out or underweighted—not only the real property itself, but also the intrinsic strength of the residents and the traditional institutions of their communities—alters the rules of the game, he said. "When people know they have value and know their price, they can start to make demands that can change the way the market frames them. It changes the assumptions we are working with."

An early step in that process is to share action-empowering data. "We give people the evidence that they're being discriminated against," says Perry. And while that information can be dispiriting, it can also spark a conversation about how best "to add value to individuals and to places where value has been extracted."

Policy options that can animate the housing market in devalued areas include tailored loan products and strategies to promote homeownership for long-term renters. To complement place-based investments, Perry urges that investments be made in people. "The places are devalued because people are devalued," he says. "We also need to restore value to individuals." Microloans, tax credits, and "baby bonds"—savings accounts started at a child's birth for families without assets—are tools to do that.

"At some point, we have to stop blaming people and start going to policies," he warns. "Many of the policies that created segregation were based on race, and when you do not address race, you don't get resolution. And so we are looking at race-based policies."

A Final Word

Stories of success and transformation offer a counterweight to the many inequitable practices documented in this chapter. Drawing on six case studies and 30 expert interviews, an Urban Institute research report considers what is needed to sustain, expand, and replicate strategies to integrate health and housing.[22] Among other key attributes, the report highlights the importance of identifying a diverse set of allies, integrating datasets, and especially engaging the community.

> *Integrating community engagement practices into program design and organizational structure increases the likelihood that projects will be embraced by the community, empowers people to take ownership of a solution, and increases trust between residents and health and housing partners.*—Urban Institute report

Those insights reinforce a core principle advanced by both Assata Richards and Andre Perry: Healthy housing is not only about bricks and mortar, but also about the fabric of a neighborhood.

Investing locally in under-resourced communities allows families the choice of staying in places they may have called home for years, perhaps generations, without sacrificing the opportunities found in more prosperous settings.

It is through a focus on equity that we can best understand the many forces that have given us the housing picture we see today, says the Urban Institute's Lisa Dubay. "That's what threads all of this together. We have this underfunded federal program [housing subsidies] that doesn't protect enough people. At the same time, we have this residential segregation that comes from a long history of structural racism. And then there is location, location, location. That really influences so many things—neighborhood safety and amenities, and the schools that kids are in."

Ultimately, meaningful progress on the nation's housing challenges will require a change in political will, Dubay says, urging health experts to become more forceful advocates for sound housing policy. "We need to make sure that public health's voice and our data and our knowledge is at the table to help push for fair housing and housing mobility as part of a comprehensive strategy to advance health equity."

SECTION III

RESHAPING THE CONDITIONS OF PLACES TO FOSTER RESILIENCE

In the previous part, contributors focused on systemic barriers to resilience, drilling down to look at those barriers affecting immigrants, incarcerated individuals, people with opioid use disorder, traumatized teenage girls, and residents in communities under housing stress. This part emphasizes how people remain strong and maintain a measure of hope even as they are challenged by inequitable conditions. Several of the chapters here examine natural and man-made disasters, acute stressors that reveal the baseline assets with which communities confront disasters, and remind us that recovery depends in part on the nature of the resources and capacity that precede adversity. Contributors describe how and why the phrase *community resilience* has been ushered into the lexicon of disaster management and explore the possibility that fundamental shifts in how we think about disasters, and prepare for them, can enhance long-term resilience. In firsthand accounts—the sights and sounds on the ground—the contributors share intimate, sometimes-poignant stories of community and individual efforts to promote resilience, even illustrating a point with the unexpected example of a sea turtle.

The section starts with the basics—the essential tools and resources necessary to support resilient communities—and highlights innovative approaches that help. Chapter 9, "Health Care Institutions Step Up to Support Resilient Communities," is a comprehensive look at a cross section of influential players working toward common goals. From Humana's

Bold Goal population health initiatives to the development of new patient care projects in federally qualified health centers to a unique economic and business alliance in Central Michigan, the health care, business, and insurance industries are nurturing resilience to foster a Culture of Health.

Chapter 10, "Strengthening the Response to Disasters and Trauma," opens with sketches of four pilot programs from the Gulf Research Program at the National Academies of Sciences, Engineering, and Medicine; the programs illustrate important resilience cornerstones in the face of environmental events and human-made disasters like chemical spills. Next, a look at resilience-strengthening practices introduces the concept of "neighborhood as patient," a framing that is gaining traction. Finally, a focus on inland communities reveals that these areas are not immune to the impacts of extreme weather, and a hypothetical town meeting explores citizen participation and social infrastructure as critical pathways to resilience.

Chapter 11, "Houston Comes Together After Hurricane Harvey," spotlights the conference site as it continues to recover from an unprecedented hurricane in 2017. Through the eyes of those still living amidst postdisaster recovery efforts, the chapter presents stories of heartache, compassion, resilience, and optimism from public health leaders, trauma physicians who work with children, air quality control specialists, determined residents, and philanthropists. As these contributors share their experiences of finding common understanding, they acknowledge the challenging nature of their work in a regional context of continuous environmental threats. Moreover, they suggest that their experiences might be a cautionary tale for other cities equally vulnerable to disasters.

This section concludes with a deeper look at the impacts of climate change and how higher temperatures, rising water levels, and more frequent storms intersect with health to intensify inequities. Drawing on reports from the Centers for Disease Control and Prevention, chapter 12, "The Environmental Justice Imperative," looks at what that means for health in underserved communities. Two well-known environmental justice experts then explore the racial inequity of climate change and chemical disasters, with a special emphasis on the extra burdens imposed on impoverished and minority communities. A discussion of "multisolving"—a new concept that knots climate change solutions and health benefits together—ends the chapter.

Health Care Institutions Step Up to Support Resilient Communities

Catherine M. Baase, MD, FAAFP, FACOEM, Board Chairperson, Michigan Health Improvement Alliance

Nivedita Mohanty, MD, Chief Research Officer and Director of Evidence-Based Practice, AllianceChicago

Andrew Renda, MD, MPH, Associate Vice President, Population Health, Humana, Inc.

A core Robert Wood Johnson Foundation (RWJF) principle is that building a Culture of Health and health equity requires a collaborative approach; no one party can do it alone. From insurers and providers to community organizations and businesses, from climate change scientists to social justice advocates, many influential players are pooling research and resources and drawing on local knowledge, technical expertise, and financial wherewithal to foster resilient communities and better health for all.

Insurers interested in promoting good health outcomes for their members while controlling costs are stepping up to cover social services that have historically fallen within the purview of other systems. Private, public, and nonprofit providers are testing new ways to deliver health care and, increasingly, health-related social services. All are mining the considerable member and patient databases available to them to develop and implement evidence-driven interventions to bolster social determinants of health, improve the lives of the individuals they serve, and leverage their resources more effectively. Meanwhile, businesses are joining community leaders to address population health, recognizing the impact on their own bottom lines and the regional economy.

Catherine M. Baase, Nivedita Mohanty, and Andrew Renda, *Health Care Institutions Step Up to Support Resilient Communities* In: *Community Resilience.* Edited by: Alonzo L. Plough, Oxford University Press (2021). © Robert Wood Johnson Foundation. DOI: 10.1093/oso/9780197559383.003.0011

This chapter explores the role of health care institutions in three distinct collaborations designed to reshape the health landscape. Presenting a private-sector perspective, Andrew Renda describes Humana's commitment to its Bold Goal population health initiative, which draws on community input to craft interventions that help combat food insecurity, loneliness, and more. Nivedita Mohanty explains how a network of federally qualified health centers is developing tools to help practitioners improve patient care. And in a melding of health and economic interests, Catherine M. Baase details a partnership between a health collaborative and an alliance of business and economic development leaders in Central Michigan.

A Private Health Insurer Tackles Social Determinants

Private insurers and corporations are exploring new ways to reduce social problems, be good corporate citizens, and succeed in a competitive private market. This interest has driven a concerted effort to address the social determinants of health while remaining cognizant of a business bottom line. Humana, for example, has evolved from an insurance company focused on using its resources effectively to a health company committed to advancing wellness and whole-person health among its members and in the communities in which they live. Among other examples of a growing corporate commitment to tackle root causes of poor health are United HealthCare, which was spotlighted in the third volume of the Culture of Health Series, and Michigan's THRIVE (Transforming Health Regionally in a Vibrant Economy) initiative, described further in this chapter.

After earning his medical and public health degrees, Andrew Renda returned to his hometown of Louisville, Kentucky, determined to tackle population health problems at their roots. Humana, where he now serves as associate vice president of its population health division, appealed to him because, with 16.6 million members, access to macro-level data, and substantial resources, it offered opportunities to experiment with new interventions as long as he could articulate both a clinical and business case.

Over time, Humana's clinical strategy became a population health strategy that focused on five points of influence: social determinants, behavioral health, primary care, home health, and pharmacy.

We've gone in three years from not knowing what a social determinant is to declaring it as one of the five most important ways we influence the people we serve.—Andrew Renda

Bold Steps, Bold Goal

Humana established its Bold Goal initiative in 2015 to carry out its vision for addressing Health Related Quality of Life (HRQoL), defined by the Centers for Disease Control and Prevention (CDC) as a person's perceived physical and mental health over time. Bold Goal aims for a 20 percent improvement in the health of its members by 2020 and beyond, as well as broad-based health improvements in the Bold Goal communities themselves. Renda describes Bold Goal as an inspirational, aspirational, and quantifiable philosophy and strategy.

> *If we are going to bring social determinants in from the cold and not relegate them to philanthropy only, we really need to start treating social determinants as clinical gaps in care.*—Andrew Renda

Some early questions shaped the approach:

- **What does 20 percent improvement in health mean?** Renda and his team concluded it meant improvements in HRQoL, which combines members' own assessments of the quality of their health with clinical data from their medical records. As research guided by Carol Graham and other contributors demonstrates (see chapter 2: "Data and Lived Experiences Both Inform Well-Being"), there is much to be learned by asking people about the circumstances of their lives.
- **What is a good measure of HRQoL?** CDC's Healthy Days tool rose to the top of the list. It asks respondents how many days, over the past 30s, they did not feel physically well, mentally well, or had to limit their activities due to physical or mental health problems. "These are simple questions that anyone can answer because they know what good health means for them," said Renda.
- The Healthy Days tool serves three functions in guiding Humana's work. First, it is used for population surveillance—about 200,000 randomly selected Humana members use the tool each year, providing both a snapshot and a trend line. Second, it is used as a leading outcome measure to evaluate interventions. And finally, it has become a proactive intervention tool—Healthy Days surveys are administered to select new Humana members, and anyone who reports more than 20 unhealthy days in a month receives a follow-up call from a Humana health navigator.
- **What can Humana do to impact HRQoL?** Research findings from an analysis that combined the Humana Healthy Days tool with RWJF County Health Rankings & Roadmaps data led to a focus on addressing loneliness and food insecurity, two factors associated with the largest impact on HRQoL.

Renda recalls telling Humana's executives, "We want you to invest in interventions around food insecurity and we need to make people less lonely." Backed with evidence demonstrating that the one in eight Americans who are food insecure are more likely to develop diabetes and cardiovascular disease, and that being lonely is more harmful than being obese or smoking 15 cigarettes a day, his team secured their eager support.

How Bold Goal Works

Bold Goal operates in communities with defined clinical and social needs, as well as a critical mass of Humana members, staff, and community partner relationships. Early phases have focused on Humana's more than four million Medicare Advantage members. As of June 2020, there were 16 Bold Goal communities throughout the United States.

Each community develops its own Bold Goal initiative within a framework that includes community meetings to build collaboration; targeted interventions, often starting with a pilot project followed by a randomized control trial; development of tools, advanced analytics, models, and evidence; and then integration and scaling.

The underlying premise of the work is that "health is local," a lesson that Renda learned in Bold Goal's early days. At first, he acknowledges, the team depended too much on Humana data and not enough on local priorities. He summarizes early community feedback: "We heard, number one, 'that is not right.' Number two, 'you didn't consult with us.' And number three, 'you don't have the right people at the table.' "

Humana now starts each project with a community meeting so the company can learn about community priorities and residents can learn about Humana's resources. An advisory board of local Humana, business, nonprofit, and public stakeholders guides each Bold Goal project.

Some interventions, such as health screenings conducted by Humana staff, are available to all residents in a community. Others, such as meal delivery, are targeted to Humana members through their coverage plans. "We have more access to and an obligation to support our members, but we need to think about how to impact the entire community as well," Renda said, pointing out that advisory boards are particularly helpful in that realm.

Tackling Food Insecurity

Responses to the 2016 Healthy Days survey indicated that Humana members who screened positive for food insecurity had an average of 27 unhealthy days each month, compared with 14.2 unhealthy days for food-secure members. With this information, and evidence that food-insecure people are 50 percent more likely to develop diabetes and 60 percent more likely to have a heart attack, both significant cost burdens on health systems, the partners moved quickly.

Humana developed a series of advanced analytic tools, including predictive models that identify people with food insecurity, loneliness, and other problems. In 2019, its clinicians and other staff conducted more than one million screenings. Humana also worked with Feeding America to create "Food Insecurity and Health: A Toolkit for Physicians and Health Care Organizations." In one local effort, the South Florida Bold Goal launched a randomized trial of a "high-tech, high-touch" intervention that included food distribution and case management.

Renda is working with the National Quality Forum, a nonprofit organization that establishes health care measures and standards, to codify food insecurity as a health quality indicator. By developing measures similar to those used for chronic conditions, that effort is an important step toward addressing social determinants as clinical best practices, he said.

Bold Goal in San Antonio

Humana has a long history in San Antonio, insuring more than 500,000 residents as of November 2019. A 2014 report of the health and fitness of the 50 largest metropolitan areas in the United States ranked San Antonio 45th, highlighting high rates of diabetes and obesity.

Through focus groups, community meetings, and a two-day "clinical town hall," residents realized that many resources were available in San Antonio, but that too few people knew about them and they were not coordinated. Bold Goal started by enhancing existing interventions.

A local Humana representative and a community leader co-chair the Bold Goal advisory board, and annual clinical town halls provide opportunities for residents to contribute and learn. One key initiative is the Diabetes Resources Guide, an interactive website that helps doctors and patients select an appropriate diabetes management program. Another is a partnership between a food bank and a Humana-owned multisite primary care physician group, which is designed to increase the availability of food distribution sites and cooking and exercise classes.

Early outcomes show promise: Between 2015 and 2018, reported unhealthy days among Humana members in San Antonio dropped by 9.8 percent, nearly halfway to the 20 percent goal.

Addressing Loneliness Among Older Adults

Humana members who suffered from loneliness had 24.4 unhealthy days per month. Between 2016 and 2019, Bold Goal activities to reduce loneliness included a "test-and-learn" project to test the feasibility of physician-administered loneliness screenings; outreach to 100,000 Humana members who reported more than 20 unhealthy days, using results to create a predictive model of members most at risk for loneliness; creation of a "Loneliness & Social Isolation Toolkit"; and incorporating loneliness screening into Humana's home care and pharmacy programs.

In partnership with other organizations, Humana is also researching and scaling promising community interventions. One connects college students to older adults, and another connects health coaches to Humana members. A targeted SilverSneakers® program provides free access to fitness centers to promote both physical activity and social interaction.

The Business Case for Investing in Social Determinants

Echoing the themes of another chapter (see chapter 14: "Investing in Social Determinants: Fresh Perspectives on the Returns"), Renda underscores the importance of both a financial payoff for the company and a clinical benefit "in order for investments in population health and social services to be sustainable."

Humana sees potential cost savings through improvements in HRQoL (better Healthy Day scores); clinical outcomes (better medication adherence, improved blood test scores); and utilization patterns (reduced time in the hospital, less use of other costly services).

> *We want to move from an insurance company with elements of health to a health company with elements of insurance, and Bold Goal is our guiding light.*—Andrew Renda

Another of Renda's goals is to align social and medical risk scores. With predictive models able to pinpoint both types of risk and the overlap between them, he sees the potential to risk adjust for both clinical and social needs and to triage resources more efficiently. Other priorities are to add new Bold Goal communities and extend Bold Goal to Medicaid, military, and privately insured members.

Engaging Community Health Centers

As insurers commit to paying more attention to social determinants of health, comparable efforts are taking hold in many clinical settings as well. One approach has its origins in the 1997 decision of four Chicago-area federally qualified health centers to pool resources and achieve economies of scale in order to develop and share innovative service delivery strategies. Eventually, the group of centers, now known as AllianceChicago, decided to invest in health information technology and pilot an electronic health record system.

The success of the shared electronic health record model, propelled forward by additional investments from the federal Health Resources and Services Administration (HRSA; the primary funder of federally qualified health centers), caught the interest of health centers across the country. By 2019, AllianceChicago had grown into a collaborative network that included more than 50 health centers in 19 states.

Research and Quality Improvement

The health information technology infrastructure afforded by the network's common electronic health record system offers robust clinical data to inform research. That database, says AllianceChicago's chief research officer, Nivedita Mohanty, provides information about "the safety net population served by the health centers and is very useful for quality improvement and research activities." For example, the database can be used to track health center performance on immunizations, cancer screenings, and other clinical measures used by HRSA's Uniform Data System, a reporting system designed to provide standardized information on federally qualified health centers.

More than 30 research partnerships with academic institutions, government agencies, private research organizations, and foundations have also helped AllianceChicago build and share knowledge. One product has been a package of clinical decision support tools that allow providers to incorporate evidence-based care into their practices. Researchers are studying how these tools are being adopted and what impact they have on care. While the tools were designed to serve members of the AllianceChicago network, they have been more broadly disseminated and are being adapted to other electronic medical record systems.

Research Questions

Mohanty describes several research questions that have been investigated through the AllianceChicago database:

- **What factors are associated with children who seek acute care at their primary medical home, rather than at a hospital emergency department?** The goal was to identify modifiable factors that could be incorporated into practice so that non-emergency acute care could be more consistently delivered within the patient's medical home, reinforcing continuity.

- **How are we using reproductive life plans in primary care?** The idea is to capture the intention to become pregnant more clearly in the health record so that health services can be delivered accordingly. This also creates opportunities to reduce maternal and child mortality and morbidity.
- **How can we build health information technology tools to identify children with hypertension?** Specific blood pressure readings are considered markers of hypertension in adults, but diagnosing children is more complex and requires an algorithm that factors in age, gender, and height.

The AllianceChicago database has also been used to help develop and assess chronic disease interventions, such as smoking cessation, cancer care coordination, obesity prevalence, and factors affecting people living with HIV.

Building Health Center Research Capacity

Community health centers often serve low-income populations, including racial and ethnic minorities, immigrants, and refugees, groups that are often excluded from health research. That exclusion, notes Mohanty, results in "missed opportunities to have treatments that are tailored to underserved populations." To mitigate this omission, AllianceChicago staff has made a concerted effort to build research capacity at the health center level, "enhancing the ability for frontline clinicians and even patients to be more active participants in all phases of the research process."

Some 29 health centers within the AllianceChicago network engage in various research activities, from contributing to large, secondary data analyses to participating in capacity-building exercises (e.g., training to write grant proposals) to implementing interventions that can be evaluated.

> We love it when we hear of research questions that are generated from frontline health center staff: nurses, providers, medical assistants who are observing something in their daily practice within the community.—Nivedita Mohanty

Partnering to Improve Care

Mohanty highlighted three programs that used analytical research to improve care for health center patients.

Tailoring Diabetes Screening Guidelines

The U.S. Preventive Services Task Force develops broad-based diabetes screening guidelines, but these may not reflect the risk profile of the population typically served by the health centers. Clinicians partnered with an academic researcher at Northwestern University Feinberg School of Medicine to ana- lyze community health data and found that individuals from certain racial and ethnic minority groups tend to have abnormal blood sugars at younger ages and lower body mass index (BMI), possibly due to variations in genetic and social factors. "Waiting to screen until the recommended ages might put those patients at a disadvantage in controlling their blood sugars at an earlier stage," Mohanty says.

AllianceChicago staff disseminated these findings to health center staff, highlighting the need to be more vigilant with certain populations. Many of the centers caring for high-risk groups have adopted new procedures, asking more questions about family history and lifestyle and factoring race, ethnicity, and cultural background into their screening criteria. These processes have helped direct patients who might not have been identified under previous protocols to diabetes prevention programs. If prediabetes is found through screening, early lifestyle modifications can change the disease trajectory and improve outcomes.

In a separate project, fellows from the Data Science for Social Good program at the University of Chicago are constructing a predictive algorithm for diabetes risk. The hope is to embed the algorithm into AllianceChicago's population health management tool to identify patients who should be screened.

Preventing Childhood Lead Poisoning

The Chicago Department of Health spearheaded a prevention-focused partner- ship with AllianceChicago, Data Science for Social Good, the City of Chicago, and the Chicago public schools to reduce lead poisoning. The goal, says Mohanty, was to "change the current dynamic of detecting lead in children from being reactive—screening kids for lead, finding they've been poisoned, then doing lead remediation [in their homes]—to being proactive." The concept was to use a predictive algorithm to locate geographic areas where lead was likely to be present and send household kits or inspectors to identify remediation actions *before* a child is poisoned.

The project was supported by RWJF; the project focused on children under age one and on pregnant women.

In developing the algorithm, the team was especially attentive to areas of both high lead prevalence and "very low child opportunity." The child oppor- tunity index, created by the city's Department of Health, uses data on social determinants of health, such as education, poverty, and employment, to identify neighborhoods where "kids are challenged at achieving their maximum poten- tial in terms of education and success," says Mohanty.

AllianceChicago, which contributed data to help build the algorithm, has implanted it as a clinical decision support tool. With a click of a button, the electronic health record generates a risk analysis, based on a child's address, and a recommendation whether the home should be inspected for lead. The provider is also able to connect by phone with the city agency that conducts inspections to request an assessment.

As of October 2019, the project was in the pilot phase. One health center has gone live, with plans to evaluate use of the tool, lead levels in children, and the findings from lead inspections. (See chapter 14: "Investing in Social Determinants: Fresh Perspectives on the Returns" for more research on the payback of lead remediation.)

Linking Health Centers and Community Resources

With development support from the Center for Medicare and Medicaid Innovation, AllianceChicago partnered with a researcher from the University of Chicago to create an online platform linked to the electronic health record, which matches the health needs of patients in real time to services available in their local area. Much of the legwork to populate the list of community assets for the CommunityRx system, as it is called, was done by a group of local youth from MAPSCorps employed as "community data scientists." Based on patient zip codes, the site identifies assets such as foot examinations available at low cost to someone with diabetes, opticians who offer free eye examinations, grocery stores that sell fresh produce, and opportunities for exercise.

A platform has been commercialized through a Chicago-based company, NowPow, which offers the tool to health systems, health plans, child welfare agencies, and networks that serve other populations. An evaluation of the initial project has shown positive results: The system generated over 250,000 personalized "HealtheRxs" (individual "prescriptions" for local services) for more than 113,000 participants during the first three years. Some 83 percent of recipients found the HealtheRx to be "very useful," and 19 percent went to a place it suggested.[1] Further evaluation is planned as health center use data become available.

Reaping the Benefits of Multisector Partnerships

As these efforts suggest, AllianceChicago's multilayered partnerships have been a great advantage to the health centers in its network, according to Mohanty, enabling them "to provide comprehensive services to patients and to be culturally responsive to their needs." Aligning research with the focus of individual health centers allows findings to be readily "implanted" in their work.

Partners who share the same core commitment to meet local needs, including academic medical centers, payers, and foundations, have been especially important to the work.

Partnerships amongst provider groups and individual providers and patients are core, but what's helped us advance our purpose is to have the multi-sectorial partnerships.—Nivedita Mohanty

Thriving in Central Michigan

Central Michigan, like many other struggling rustbelt communities in the Midwest, faces significant health and economic challenges. "When we looked at the last 15 years, it was not a pretty picture," says Catherine M. Baase, a long-time resident and area leader. Noting job and population losses and high poverty rates, Baase concludes, "We can't do something small here; we need something extraordinary."

THRIVE, a collaboration of health, business, and community leaders, aims to be that "something extraordinary."[2] THRIVE has two clear goals: improved health and sustained economic growth throughout the 14-county region of Central Michigan. Baase, a physician who served as the Dow Chemical Company's chief health officer and global director of health services for more than 20 years, is well positioned to steer the region toward those goals.

Business and Health, Two Systems or One?

An essential first step toward improving population health and strengthening the local economy, Baase concludes, is to help business leaders connect the dots between individual and community health and business success.

The business community is often not conscious of the business case for health, but even when they do understand it, they think of health as a morass that is undiscernible, and they hope and pray that somebody might be figuring it out.—Catherine M. Baase

Baase's value proposition starts with the obvious: Businesses want to fuel consumer purchases and economic growth. When a disproportionate share of private resources is diverted to medical expenses, less money is available for marketplace goods and other business priorities. "By syphoning money into health care costs, we undermine the foundational elements of business success, including critical items like education and infrastructure," Baase says.

Business success is tied to health in ways that go beyond profitability, however. Employees who are not healthy are less able to concentrate or move about with ease. Feeling poorly or under stress, they are more likely to be injured, absent, or unmotivated. Businesses located in communities with poor health indicators typically find it harder to find skilled, reliable workers.

THRIVE, established in 2017, is built on the conviction that business is advantaged when the population is healthy, and health is advantaged when the economic environment is strong. It is jointly governed by the Michigan Health Improvement Alliance, a nonprofit collaborative aimed at improving health and health delivery in Central Michigan, where Baase serves as the board chair, and the Great Lakes Bay Regional Alliance, which brings together business and economic development leaders in the region.

A Transformational Kind of Change

Two early insights shaped THRIVE's commitment to transformational change. First, small programs are not transformative, so scale became a significant criterion. Scale also "meant we would have to address sustainability," Baase recognizes. Second, transformational work succeeds only if it gets to root causes and rests on a solid foundation of principles and protocols. Without that foundation, it becomes too easy for those involved to seize on new ideas simply because they sound promising, regardless of their broader context.

> We were tired and discouraged by not seeing improved outcomes from all the work we had been doing. So, we needed a transformational kind of change. It couldn't be small.—Catherine M. Baase

With guidance from both the Michigan and the Great Lakes Bay Regional Alliance, community members spent the summer of 2017 interviewing many dozens of people. Results indicated readiness for this transformational work. Many community leaders were convened to develop a detailed ecosystem map reflecting regional drivers, relationships, opportunities, and obstacles. A THRIVE portfolio was created from the mapping, with teams of 10–12 people exploring levers to advance five priorities:

- Improve preventive care and mental health and well-being.
- Enhance the attraction of the region as a place to live and work.
- Create jobs.

- Expand provider capacity through professional education and pipeline development.
- Invest in the whole community to reduce barriers by addressing social determinants.

The teams then worked within a structured charter to inventory ongoing initiatives in each priority area, identify and catalog evidence-based interventions, and develop recommendations for action.

A 2017 decision to employ the ReThink Health Dynamics simulation model turned out to be "an extraordinary adder to the business case and a huge boost to momentum," Baase says. The model explores "alternative interventions to improve and transform health and health care at a local level—the level of a city, county, health service region, or state."[3] The simulation made it possible to project the likely impacts and outcomes of an initial set of 34 THRIVE interventions through 2040 compared to business-as-usual scenarios. Key findings are shown in the table:

Indicator	Business as Usual	THRIVE
Population	30,000-person population loss	20,000-person population gain
Workforce	25,000-person workforce loss	18,000-person workforce gain
Economic status	33.4% disadvantaged	22.3% disadvantaged
Salaries and wages	Salaries and wages stagnate	Salaries and wages grow 8%

The simulation also found that with THRIVE, 60,000 more people would receive commercial health insurance and 40,000 fewer would need Medicaid. In addition, 40,000 fewer people would engage in high-risk behaviors, even as the population grows.

Building on the simulation findings, THRIVE focused on eight interventions for its first implementation phase. These include establishing regional focus on attracting innovative industries and entrepreneurs; creating a regional health education hub; and educating stakeholders about trauma-informed care for vulnerable children. The opioid epidemic is also a focus; that intervention expands the use of nonpharmacological approaches to pain, such as meditation and acupuncture, which is an identified gap in services.

Evaluation and Financing for Sustainability

The multitiered evaluation of the THRIVE strategy starts with the dual endpoints of improved health and economic growth. Drilling down, the evaluation measures health impact, health care system and provider impact, and economic impact, with a sequence of increasingly specific metrics in each area.

Securing adequate long-term financing is a key priority for 2020. To plan for sustainability, the partner alliances have created a master list of more than 14 potential financing sources, including grants, loans, impact investments, pay-for-success strategies, Medicaid and community development funds, tax incentives, and earned income. The plan is to match each intervention with potential financing mechanisms, document likely costs and revenue, and establish a work plan and timeline.

In 2019, community leaders demonstrated their commitment to THRIVE by contributing nearly $1 million in capacity funding to support three years of development. These funds allowed THRIVE to move beyond relying on volunteers and retain a portfolio director, a chief health and chief economic officer, and other staff.

Reflections on THRIVE

THRIVE started with a big vision; the framework and structure followed soon after. "The decision to think and act together and boldly was a big success. If we hadn't committed to that end, we would be nowhere," Baase says.

She reflected on three of the many lessons to emerge.

- **Smart decisions:** THRIVE would not have come as far as it has without a commitment to absolute transparency and open communication, engagement of the business community, grasping the importance of building financing mechanisms, and securing the commitment of volunteers.
- **Integrator agencies:** The Michigan Health Improvement Alliance and Great Lakes Bay Regional Alliance, with their long-term operations in the community, provide a critical anchor for THRIVE. Both organizations leveraged their credibility to secure and sustain extensive volunteer resources in THRIVE's first two years. Their data repositories and program inventories provided the groundwork on which THRIVE priority teams could build, as well as baseline data for the evaluation.
- **Progress over perfection:** Striking the balance between addressing urgent problems and taking time to plan is an ongoing constructive tension. At times, Baase finds it hard to act before comprehensive and sophisticated planning has been done, yet she recognizes that "things can't always be perfect.

We have to keep moving and decide to address urgency with a prudent course and expediency."

A Final Word

The initiatives described in this chapter underscore the need for many types of organizations to play important roles in building a Culture of Health and health equity. They demonstrate that a large organization can expand its view of what constitutes health and well-being; that clinical research can engage often-overlooked populations as partners in research studies; and that health improvement and economic growth are compatible, indeed mutually reinforcing, goals—all important lessons for others coming together to improve health and well-being in both local communities and across wide regions.

As these experiences highlight strategies to improve individual and community health, they also remind us of the power of collaboration. They offer models that can help meet community needs when resources are scarce—especially important when persistent disaster threats are intensified by the coronavirus pandemic. During a period that requires an unprecedented degree of resilience, American society must leverage the expertise, enthusiasm, and commitment of multisectoral leaders and organizations with deep community experience.

10

Strengthening the Response to Disasters and Trauma

Joie D. Acosta, PhD, Senior Behavioral/Social Scientist, RAND Corporation

Lauren Alexander Augustine, PhD, Executive Director, Gulf Research Program, the National Academies of Sciences, Engineering, and Medicine (National Academies)

Traci L. Birch, PhD, AICP, Managing Director, Louisiana State University Coastal Sustainability Studio

Elka Gotfryd, MS, Principal and Consultant, Gotfryd Group Inc.

Lourdes J. Rodríguez, DrPH, Senior Program Officer, St. David's Foundation

Sheila B. Savannah, MA, Managing Director, Prevention Institute

Benjamin Springgate, MD, MPH, Director of the Center for Healthcare Value and Equity, Chief of Community and Population Medicine, Louisiana State University Health Sciences Center-New Orleans

Is there a formula for community resilience?

Answering this question is at once complex and urgent, primarily for two reasons. First, the drive to build resilient communities is typically born of the need to respond to adverse situations: Consider community resilience in the aftermath of environmental and human-made crises like hurricanes, flooding, oil spills, wildfires, and violence, or community resilience in the face of historic disparities in employment, health, education, and housing. Second, communities across the United States are increasingly vulnerable to severe disasters and widening inequity.

Joie D. Acosta, Lauren Alexander Augustine, Traci L. Birch, Elka Gotfryd, Lourdes J. Rodríguez, Sheila B. Savannah, and Benjamin Springgate, *Strengthening the Response to Disasters and Trauma* In: *Community Resilience*. Edited by: Alonzo L. Plough, Oxford University Press (2021). © Robert Wood Johnson Foundation. DOI: 10.1093/oso/9780197559383.003.0012

Community resilience has been a part of the country's dialogue over the past decade, long before the COVID-19 pandemic surfaced globally in 2020. According to a 2019 report by the National Academies of Sciences, Engineering, and Medicine (National Academies), a body of research and programming has emerged to inform resilience at both the individual and global levels, incorporating everything from infrastructure to ecosystems to health.[1] These efforts have borne fruit with their insights about what it takes to nurture resilience.

While previous chapters highlighted services and supports that foster resilience, this one looks in depth at the science of healthy communities and the study of resilience within a community framework—a key principle in the commitment of the Robert Wood Johnson Foundation (RWJF) to building a national Culture of Health. Throughout this chapter, it becomes abundantly clear that existing conditions before disasters strike have an enormous influence on what happens afterward. Stressors such as poor housing, poverty, and segregation in flood-prone coastal communities are often as determinant as the storm itself. As disaster-related research often documents, a heightened focus on pre- and peridisaster community conditions can have enormous influence on how a community's health is impacted by acute events.[2]

This chapter opens with the Gulf Research Program's Lauren Alexander Augustine, who presents four pilot programs from around the country that illustrate the cornerstones of community resilience. Next, Benjamin Springgate, who directs the Center for Health Care Value and Equity at Louisiana State University Health Sciences Center–New Orleans, examines resilience as a reflection of individual communities and describes a research network that promotes research on resilience-strengthening practices. Lourdes J. Rodríguez, from the University of Texas at Austin, and Prevention Institute's Sheila B. Savannah then explain how neighborhoods that are striving for resilience should be involved like patients in the process of healing.

Finally, in two Spotlights at the end of the chapter, contributors offer unique perspectives on resilient communities. Traci L. Birch looks at why resilience efforts should also focus on inland communities that are no longer immune to the impacts of climate change and extreme weather ("Spotlight: Inland From the Coast, Resilience Efforts Follow the Water"). And Joie D. Acosta and Elka Gotfryd encourage us to think broadly about resilience as they explore opportunities to build responsive social infrastructure through engaged citizen participation ("Spotlight: Social Infrastructure as a Pathway to Resilience").

In many ways, the devastation of Hurricane Katrina was a turning point for understanding and managing disasters. . . . It brought the phrase

"community resilience" into the lexicon of disaster management.—National
Academies of Sciences, Engineering, Medicine, 2019 report on community resilience[3]

What We Know About Community
Resilience: Four Examples

A string of devastating disasters over the past decade had a single consolation—
It offered important lessons about building resilient communities.

When Hurricane Katrina hit the Gulf Coast and New Orleans in 2005, the ca-
lamitous storm exposed a deadly combination of existing community stressors
and aging infrastructure. It also spawned a new vocabulary that spoke to the
need to prepare for disasters, not merely to respond to them. In 2009, federal
spending on disaster relief soared to $1.4 billion, a dramatic increase over the
$20.9 million spent in 1953 and "one indicator of the urgent need to increase the
nation's resilience," declared the National Academies in a 2012 report, "Disaster
Resilience: A National Imperative."[4]

Five years after Katrina, the Deepwater Horizon oil spill and explosion in the
Gulf of Mexico occurred in the same region, renewing questions about resilience in the states and communities bordering the Gulf Coast. By 2011, multiple
disasters—including 14 related to weather and climate—caused the deaths of
nearly 600 people, displaced thousands more, and created more than $55 billion
in economic damages across the United States, "breaking all records since these
data were first reported in 1980," according to the report.[5]

Lauren Alexander Augustine was in charge of resilience programs at the
National Academies as these incidents unfolded. She and the people around her
understood that the nation's approach to disasters—which relied heavily on after-
the-fact responses—was no longer sustainable. "Everyone wanted to know, 'How
do you look at this differently?'" she says. Data already suggested that the cost of
disasters would continue to escalate both in dollar terms and in social, cultural, and
environmental losses; that given the population's shift toward coastal and southern
regions, more people would be impacted by hurricanes, drought, and floods; and
that at-risk populations, including people who were aging or poor, would need
more help as infrastructure and services were taxed beyond their capacity.

Disaster Resilience: A National Imperative

The National Academies disaster resilience report, released more than seven
years after Hurricane Katrina, left no doubt that embracing preparedness as a
shared responsibility was the only way forward.

As the report stated, "If our nation continues its current approach to disasters—one that relies heavily on responding to them after they occur—the toll taken by disasters will likely continue to rise. We can choose instead to embark on a new path, one that recognizes the value of resilience to the individual, household, community, and nation."

A culture of resilience provides a way to reduce vulnerability to disasters and their impacts before they occur, with the potential to decrease disasters' costs and consequences.—"Disaster Resilience," 2012

The report broadly outlined four principles for building a resilient community, cornerstones that essentially defined disaster resilience as a shared responsibility among citizens, the private sector, and government[6]:

- **Build and strengthen coalitions and partnerships across sectors:** Federal, state, and local governments should support the creation and maintenance of broad-based coalitions to build resilience at local and regional levels. Though communities vary greatly, some basic premises apply to them all:
  - Essential services, such as health, education, and public and private infrastructure, need to be robust.
  - Individuals and groups need to know about risks and how to reduce them.
  - Communities, neighborhoods, and families need to be organized to prepare for disasters.
  - Land-use planning needs to be sound.
  - Appropriate building codes and standards need to be adopted and enforced.
- **Understand, communicate, and manage risk:** The public and private sectors in a community should work cooperatively on a risk management strategy that includes tools to reduce or spread risk.
- **Measure resilience and track progress:** Federal agencies should incorporate national resilience as a guiding principle to inform their mission, actions, and the programs and policies they support at all levels.
- **Share data, tools, and best practices:** A national repository of disaster-related data should be established to document injuries, loss of life, property loss, and impacts on economic activity. And there is a need for federal agencies, state and local partners, and professional groups to develop metrics or measurements of resilience that would help cities and local governments improve disaster preparedness and reduce their risks.

Although disasters will continue to occur, actions that move the nation from a reactive to a proactive approach will reduce the societal and economic burdens and impacts that disasters cause. . . . The reward for our efforts will be a safer, healthier, more secure, and more prosperous nation.—"Disaster Resilience," 2012

Four Communities, Four Paths to Resilience, Four Surprises

The "Disaster Resilience" report was so well received that the National Academies asked Augustine to implement and test its findings—a highly unusual step in an organization whose research findings are typically tested by other groups. Toward this goal, Augustine and her team started a new pilot program at the National Academies called ResilientAmerica, which partnered with four communities: Charleston, South Carolina; Cedar Rapids, Iowa; Tulsa, Oklahoma; and the Seattle/Greater Puget Sound region of Washington State.[7]

Augustine packaged the study's four tenets and presented them to these communities. "We basically said if you want to have resilience, you have to understand your risk to better manage it. You have to measure your resilience. If you're going to make investments in your community, you have to figure out if you're making any progress towards a return on those investments. And then the last thing, if you learn something you should share what you learn. We created pilot programs, and wow, were we surprised."

No One Wanted to Talk About Disasters

The four communities agreed to participate in ResilientAmerica beginning in 2014, but as Augustine soon learned, "They didn't want to talk about disasters." Augustine was not only surprised but also confused. "As we entered into the conversations with these communities, the title said, 'disaster resilience.' It was pretty clear. But instead of talking about disasters, they wanted to talk about things like at-risk populations, those who were the most disenfranchised. Because in each community, if you can't bring along those who are already on the margins, you're not moving along at all. And they also wanted to talk about economic resilience; if you have no livelihood in this community, you don't have a community."

(Notably, this finding tracks with what Bernadette Hohl uncovered in chapter 3: "A New Narrative on Gun Violence" when she asked residents to talk about gun violence and they approached the topic by first talking about a clean, safe, and civil environment. A similar concept surfaces in chapter 8: "Home, the Heart of Place," where standard metrics describe a community under severe economic stress, yet residents say they are satisfied with living there. In each case, local people helped shift the assumptions and perspectives of the researchers.)

In response to her conversations, Augustine, a Harvard-trained engineer, flipped to "consequence analysis"—an engineering term that refers in this context to identifying something the community wants to avoid. In Tulsa, citizens viewed resilience through the lens of economic security—They didn't want their economic base to fail. In Charleston, stakeholders said that the economy of their vibrant, historic city would be devastated if it lost its tourists. This shift in perspective—from addressing disasters to safeguarding the financial footing—engaged the private and public sectors and proved critical to fostering community involvement.

The ResilientAmerica Results

- **Cedar Rapids, Iowa:** Since it was hit by catastrophic floods in 2008, Cedar Rapids/Linn County had made significant progress toward recovery and was continuing its efforts to build resilience against future flooding and other hazards. ResilientAmerica partnered with Cedar Rapids/Linn County in September 2014, and for the next four years explored priorities that included building on community strengths; engaging diverse voices in resilience efforts; building resilience within at-risk populations; effectively communicating risk to the public; building trust and multistakeholder, multigenerational partnerships; and developing real-time decision-making capability during a disaster.[8]

- **Charleston, South Carolina:** This southern city needed to address persistent flooding events, storm surges, earthquakes, terrorism, hazardous material incidents, hurricanes, and more—the list was remarkably long. "Charleston is subject to something like 19 different natural hazards, including the potential for earthquakes," says Augustine. "The only things Charleston isn't subject to are sandstorms and volcanoes." After focusing on flood resilience in recent years, a volunteer group of individuals representing public and private-sector organizations worked with ResilientAmerica to create the Charleston Resilience Network to share information, connect partners, and create a unified strategy. In 2015, the city identified sea-level rise as a top priority, and over the next two years, ResilientAmerica implemented a framework to measure Charleston's baseline flood resilience and the city created and filled the position of chief resilience officer.[9]

- **Central Puget Sound Region:** The Seattle/Puget Sound region faces a variety of natural hazards, including volcanoes, earthquakes, floods, and landslides, as well as the rising seas. Taking a regional focus, ResilientAmerica partnered with the Puget Sound Regional Council to explore priorities, including climate adaptation, equity, transportation, and rapid economic growth. Data collected from local jurisdictions across four counties helped spotlight the potential risks and impacts of climate change and helped these jurisdictions include climate resilience or adaptation policies in local planning.[10]

• **Tulsa, Oklahoma:** Tulsa had already developed an effective flood plan and flood control system since the epic Memorial Day flood of 1984 (in fact, Tulsa's approach has been called "a national blueprint for managing floods"[11]). When it joined ResilientAmerica in 2016, Tulsa's priority was to become economically resilient. It pursued that goal with multisector representatives who explored the potential relationship between sales tax revenue and resilience.[12]

Resilience, Racism, Sea Turtles

Augustine frequently references the need to "blur the lines" when talking about resilience and ResilientAmerica projects. Like the "ish" reference from the conference's keynote speaker Kenya Barris, the creator of the popular *Black-ish* television series (see chapter 1: "The Storytellers"), Augustine likes to think of "resilience-ish" as being agile, innovative, and able to meet community needs through a multidimensional lens.

This happened more than once in Charleston, which endured two widely publicized racial tragedies during the pilot period. In April 2015, a White police officer fatally shot an unarmed Black man who was fleeing arrest. And in June 2015, nine Black men and women were killed by a White supremacist inside an historic Black church. Initially, the city didn't want to talk about these incidents or racism any more than it wanted to talk about sea level rise or disasters, Augustine says.

That changed during a meeting, when the head of the local aquarium brought up sea turtles: "Everyone loves sea turtles," he said. Augustine was initially flummoxed by the seeming aside. "What is he talking about?" she wondered. "This is not helping."

But the local leader continued, "Everyone loves sea turtles, and everyone wants to protect their habitat. And where do the sea turtles live? They live on this membrane of water and land, where poor people live, where people of color live. And if we can talk about flooding and how to respond to the habitat of sea turtles, we get in the back door to this other question that no one really wants to talk about."

It was a profound moment for Augustine. "You can't talk about flooding resilience in Charleston without talking about who gets flooded first, the longest, who is impacted the most, whose kids are missing school because black mold is in their house and they have an asthma condition. But you can't always talk about vulnerable populations and racism in an open way so we talked about it in terms of sea turtles. It opened the entire social and natural habitat dimensions, and it was brilliant."

The whole point, Augustine realized, is to find the entry point that resonates for the community in which you are working, recognizing that the approach will likely evolve over time and perhaps build stronger community consensus along the way.

> *People have to be prepared to say, "This isn't perfect, but we will start anyway."*—Lauren Alexander Augustine

In 2018, Augustine was named executive director of the National Academies' Gulf Research Program, which is under the auspices of the National Academies of Sciences, Engineering, and Medicine. It is funded over three decades by a $500-million, Department of Justice-created endowment as part of the criminal settlements from the 2010 *Deepwater Horizon* disaster, the largest offshore oil spill in U.S. history. Through 2043, the Gulf Research Program is dedicated to enhancing healthy ecosystems, thriving communities, safer offshore energy systems, and capacity in the Gulf of Mexico and other U.S. outer-continental shelf regions.[13]

Augustine views the challenge of guiding the Gulf Research Program as "an enormous opportunity," one that parallels her work with ResilientAmerica. "I cannot begin to guess what this landscape is going to look like in 10 years, never mind 30 years," she admits. "But if we do it right, we can address so many issues that cut across economy, environment, health, and resilience. We should have an impact in this region that lives on."

Community Resilience and Mental Health

When Augustine took the lead job at the Gulf Research Program, Benjamin Springgate was one of the many scholars and practitioners already making important contributions there. But his interest in the region dates back many years.

Two months before Hurricane Katrina struck New Orleans in 2005, Springgate had completed a medical residency in the city where he grew up and started his RWJF Clinical Scholar Program fellowship at the University of California at Los Angeles (UCLA). In the months after the storm, he and his partners tracked the prevalence of mental illness among the residents impacted by Katrina, including his former neighborhood of New Orleans East, which had been devastated by flooding and storm surge. Their research—as well as the lived experiences of his former neighbors—revealed that up to 40 percent of residents had experienced potentially disabling symptoms of depression, anxiety, and post-traumatic stress disorder, and that the prevalence of mental illness in the impacted community had more than doubled.[14]

> *The ability of any community to rebuild in the face of disaster is going to be impacted substantially when such a high proportion of individuals and families are struggling just to get out of bed each day because of the emotional and mental stress they are enduring.*—Benjamin Springgate

Springgate's career was profoundly shaped by Hurricane Katrina and his experiences as a clinical scholar, and he continued to focus on populations most at risk from climate change—particularly in poor communities of color where people are impacted by structural racism and repeatedly traumatized. "Those with few financial resources, pre-existing housing insecurity, or mental health problems are more likely to bear the brunt of these consequences of climate change and disaster," he says. (For an in-depth look at the relationship between climate change, health, equity, and the exigency of resilience, see chapter 12: "The Environmental Justice Imperative.")

During his fellowship as a UCLA Clinical Scholar, Springgate returned to New Orleans and with grants from RWJF and others founded the Rapid Evaluation and Action for Community Health in New Orleans (REACH NOLA), which brought together community members, service providers, faith-based organizations, and academic institutions to address stress, depression, anxiety, and trauma-related mental illness among the city's low-income, uninsured residents.

Informed by his work at REACH NOLA and subsequent efforts of community and academic partners, Springgate and his collaborators launched C-LEARN—the Community Resilience Learning Collaborative and Research Network—in 2017. C-LEARN is part of a $10.8-million initiative jointly funded by the Gulf Research Program and RWJF to enhance the science and practice of resilience in the Gulf of Mexico region.[15,16]

C-LEARN: A Research Network to Strengthen Community Resilience

Springgate acknowledges that resilience efforts happen at individual, family, and community levels. In many ways, C-LEARN embraces all three. Today, this ongoing project strives to build on local strengths and resources to improve resilience and mental health outcomes in coastal communities in southern Louisiana. Based on a community-partnered participatory research model, C-LEARN is designed to test, measure, and promote practices that can strengthen preparedness and community resilience in disaster-prone communities.[17,18]

Granted, resilience measurement science is fairly new and, as one recent report noted, "not mature enough to clearly articulate" what approach works best in practice."[19] But through C-LEARN, a cohort of partners in Baton Rouge, New Orleans, and coastal southern Louisiana is building knowledge in two distinct phases:

- **Phase One:** Key informant interviews conducted at 47 agencies in 2018 helped to identify important themes and takeaways about community priorities related to stressors and strengths.[20]

Among the themes:
- o The changing environment in South Louisiana makes disaster resilience challenging yet critical.
- o Building partnerships among a wide variety of agencies and developing cross-sector collaborations before a disaster strikes strengthens communities' abilities to address challenges.
- o Focusing on the strengths of communities and having pride in the community helps build resilience.
- o Building and earning a community's trust can take a lot of time but is vital to providing adequate services and creating strong partnerships and resilient communities.[21]

Among the key interview takeaways[22]:
- o **Active listening fortifies resilience through understanding.** Listening actively to community members and their stories builds trust, shows understanding, and fortifies community resilience.
- o **Finances and funding impact resilience.** Obtaining and maintaining funding can be a challenging part of disaster recovery, and it is important to navigate financial systems together.
- o **Faith-based organizations serve as hubs for resilience.** Faith-based organizations often have a deep understanding of community members and can provide valuable insights about how to serve the community and offer a safe haven in times of need.[23]
- **Phase Two:** Based on these findings, Phase Two introduced new community-level and individual-level interventions and mobile technology tools. The interventions included training programs on disaster preparedness, reducing social risk factors, enhancing mental health resilience, and coalition building. The use of mobile health technology apps—one uses a "Catch it, Check it, Change it" framework—is designed to bolster resilience, provide informational resources during disasters, and help people manage stress during difficult times.[24]

While the lessons from C-LEARN about working with communities resonate with other examples in this chapter about the importance of building
trust and active listening, Springgate views C-LEARN as a unique study
for two reasons. First, it supports the integration of diverse sectors that
are usually studied separately: namely, disaster resilience, mental health,
and social determinants of health.[25] And second, it elevates the voices of
the community—what he calls the "PhDs of the sidewalks," a concept that
Springgate traces back to his mentor, Loretta Jones, of Healthy African
American Families II in Los Angeles.[26] He is hopeful that C-LEARN's
findings can be scaled and applied elsewhere, even in cities far from a
southern coastal environment.

> *If academic investigators or funders or policy makers want to see progress in*
> *achieving health equity and overcoming health disparities, then we have to look*
> *to terms and collaborations that include the PhDs of the sidewalks.*—Benjamin
> Springgate

Neighborhood as Patient: When Place Needs Healing

When it comes to building resilient communities, the ResilientAmerica
and C-LEARN projects highlight the importance of forging community-
research partnerships by developing relationships, eliciting citizen input, and
building trust before disaster strikes. (Citizen participation in creating resilient communities is examined further in "Spotlight: Social Infrastructure as
a Pathway to Resilience," and the importance of resilient inland communities
is described in "Spotlight: Inland From the Coast," both at the end of this
chapter.)

But what happens when a community or a neighborhood is plagued by
trauma long before a single catastrophic event occurs? What happens when
neighborhoods are traumatized by long-standing poverty and historically inadequate access to resources like education, health care, safe housing, and employment opportunities? In short, what does building resilience look like when the
neighborhood is the patient and the place needs healing?

These are the questions posed by Lourdes J. Rodríguez and Sheila B. Savannah,
who took accepted principles of resilience and its challenges and reframed them
through a concept they call "neighborhood as patient."

"We think of neighborhoods in a utopian way, as cohesive places where people
align around specific issues, where everybody may share the same aspects of vulnerability," says Rodríguez. "And that's not always the case."

A Neighborhood's Social Capital

Rodríguez has a theory: The neighborhood is where we make deposits into social capital accounts, and access to these assets depends on neighborhood characteristics and connections. Social capital is accrued through engagement, social networks, neighborliness, community supports, and sense of security and safety. If those features are missing, the social capital account is basically empty, which compromises a neighborhood's ability to be resilient.

Rodríguez argues that it is imperative to create neighborhood connections where they are missing. "When we stop investing in our neighborhoods, we isolate, separate, sort people out in ways that limit our ability to make connections," she notes.

Rodríguez posits that a healthy neighborhood has three basic layers: a physical component (i.e., good housing stock); a social component (inclusive, with opportunities to connect to others); and an economic component (entities that provide basic services, like grocery stores, day care, and health clinics). "For me, community is a collective unit—'collective' because it brings together more than one individual, but a 'unit' because members of the collective are seen as part of a complex whole."

> *Community power is the opportunity granted to collectives when we realize that together we can achieve more than we could individually. The more power we accrue, the more resilient we are as a community—and that helps us withstand threats to the collective.*—Lourdes J. Rodríguez

THRIVE: The Tool for Health and Resilience in Vulnerable Environments

The symptoms of community trauma do not always become headlines. Sometimes, it is the broken glass in the playground or the boarded-up row houses and factory buildings that do the harm. It may be a low-income inner-city housing unit that faces a parking lot instead of green space or a crumbling shack with a partially exposed roof in a rural community. The abandoned corner grocery store, the shuttered library, the bus stop shelter covered in negative graffiti also are symptoms that signal the need for healing.

According to Prevention Institute, a national nonprofit devoted to integrating prevention and health equity into policy and practice, these snapshots of community trauma reflect chronic adversity. They speak to a systemic lack of equitable opportunities, a deteriorating built environment, and the resulting erosion of solid social and cultural assets. Such community determinants undermine a Culture of Health as they foster disconnected and damaged social networks,

elevate destructive norms, and promote a low sense of political and social effi-
cacy among residents.[27]

Yet these images can also be an inspiration for promoting change, believes
Sheila B. Savannah, who is managing director of Prevention Institute.

*If you look at these pictures and ask yourself "Where is the strength?" that's how
you begin to help communities connect to their strengths, their capabilities, their
potential. Because therein lies the ability to begin to heal trauma and begin to
create change.*—Sheila B. Savannah

Prevention Institute's Tool for Health & Resilience in Vulnerable Environments
(THRIVE)[28] was created to answer the question, "What can communities do
to improve health and safety and promote health equity?" As both a tool and a
framework to help traumatized communities begin to heal, it identifies 12 community determinants of health and safety in three, interrelated clusters: social-
cultural environment (people); the physical/built environment (place); and the
economic/educational environment (equitable opportunity).[29]

THRIVE is used to help communities "think and move upstream" as they
assess local health determinants, prioritize them, and take action to change their
surroundings to improve health, safety, and health equity. THRIVE also helps
communities inform policy and program directions for local, state, and national
initiatives. The tool can be used by a wide range of neighborhoods that need
healing, including communities impacted by hurricanes, neighborhoods dealing
with racial discrimination, and regions dealing with opioid epidemics.

Community resilience, concludes Savannah, "is the ability and capacity
of a community to adapt, recover, and thrive, even in the face of adversity—
especially prolonged adversity."

*The most precious part of community resilience is engagement. Because just like
an individual patient, if a community is not engaged in setting the course for
their healing it is not going to happen.*—Sheila B. Savannah

A Final Word

The National Academies' 2012 disaster resilience report presented a vision of
what a more resilient America would look like in 2030. According to the report,
it would be a place where the following apply[30] :

- Information on the risks and vulnerabilities that individuals and communities face is transparent and easily accessible by all.
- All levels of government, communities, and the private sector have designed
  resilience strategies and operation plans based on that information.

- Proactive investments and policy decisions—including those to prepare for, mitigate, respond to, and recover from disasters—have reduced the human and economic toll of disasters.
- Community coalitions are widely organized and supported to provide essential services before and after disasters occur.
- Recovery after disasters is rapid.

Over the next decade, Augustine is hopeful that the United States will be a resilient nation that reflects these goals. She believes resilience projects slated to continue until 2043 under the Gulf Research Program will have a dramatic impact on not only the Gulf region but also all over the country. In fact, a 2019 report from the National Academies noted that the Gulf Research Program is "in a unique position to substantially advance community resilience"[31] as it becomes increasingly clear that the lessons and methods of environmental resilience illuminate our understanding of both individual and community resilience.

Springgate strikes a more somber tone, noting that while he is hopeful about the future, he also recognizes that obstacles to resilience will remain, and in some cases intensify. "Communities already threatened by climate change may disappear off the map within our lifetimes," he cautions. "In low-lying coastal communities, it is probably too late to focus on physical structures. Projections suggest that many of these communities will soon be entirely uninhabitable. The tide is rising, and the rise seems to be inexorable."

Spotlight

Inland From the Coast

Traci L. Birch, PhD, AICP, Managing Director, Louisiana State
University Coastal Sustainability Studio

*In August 2016, the city of Baton Rouge and its surrounding parishes were
inundated with more than two-and-a-half feet of rain. For perspective, that's five
times as much as the area normally gets in a month. The resulting flood caused 13
deaths, and Baton Rouge officials reported that 30,000 people had to be rescued
from homes and cars; 11,000 needed shelter; and 90,000 homes and 6,000
businesses were damaged. The Red Cross called this the "worst U.S. natural disaster since Hurricane Sandy in 2012."[1]*

*It was also, says Traci L. Birch grimly, "the most recent natural disaster in
Louisiana that nobody has ever heard of."*

*For Birch, a coastal planner by training in post-Katrina South Louisiana,
with a PhD in urban studies, the flooding is significant for another important
reason: Baton Rouge is 150 miles inland and has historically been considered safe
from the flooding that is more familiar to coastal areas like New Orleans. But recent disasters—not only in Baton Rouge, but also in Columbia, South Carolina;
Raleigh, North Carolina; and Austin, Texas—have forced researchers to recognize that risks from sea-level rise, climate change, and extreme weather threaten
floods across a much wider swath of terrain.*

There was kind of a magic line on the map where we said, "We don't have
to worry about flooding here because that's inland." And in 2016, all those
places we thought were "safe," all those places we told people to move to, they
flooded.—Traci L. Birch

*With the goal of creating a framework for restoring community well-being and
resilience, Birch now leads of team of researchers, engineers, architects, landscape
architects, policymakers, and community members to study climate change and
extreme weather responses across the greater Baton Rouge inland-coastal region.
The project, called "Inland From the Coast: A Multi-Scalar Approach to Regional*

Traci L. Birch, *Spotlight: Inland From the Coast* In: *Community Resilience*. Edited by: Alonzo L. Plough, Oxford University
Press (2021). © Robert Wood Johnson Foundation. DOI: 10.1093/oso/9780197559383.003.0013

Climate Change Responses," is one of four Gulf of Mexico community resilience projects funded jointly by the National Academies' Gulf Research Program and the Robert Wood Johnson Foundation in 2017.[2]

According to Birch, one of the key elements of the project is to "work with a community so that when we leave, they own it." Ongoing efforts in four communities in Louisiana—Baker, Denham Springs, East Baton Rouge Parish, and Ascension Parish—are designed to figure out what they need to become more resilient. The work proceeds along three research tracks—ecosystem dynamics, community well-being, and design intervention.

For example, the Baker community decided in 2019 to focus on storm water management in a comprehensive way. "It's about updating your ordinances so that you don't end up with 300 houses outside the flood area designation," says Birch. "It's about building connectivity between communities and elected officials."

Birch believes strongly in the benefits of listening to and learning from the community. "I come in assuming that the people on the ground have much more knowledge about their community than I do," she says. "People pay attention. They know when it rains really hard, they know which direction the water flows, they know what floods first. There's a subtlety in a landscape that people can share with you, if you ask them."

And though things like "green infrastructure" sound good, nobody knows what that means, right? But if we talk about parks that hold storm water, that makes sense to people.—Traci L. Birch

This current study will have wide applications for inland-coastal areas likely to become even more vulnerable to storm surges in the not-too-distant future.

Spotlight

Social Infrastructure as a Pathway to Resilience

Joie D. Acosta, PhD, Senior Behavioral/Social Scientist, RAND Corporation

Elka Gotfryd, MS, Principal and Consultant, Gotfryd Group Inc.

Everyone has heard the familiar slogan "the system is broken." In the context of community resilience, these words shed light on a deep frustration because so many of our current systems of governance fail to respond effectively to pressing societal issues. In other words, these systems generally operate in ways that do not foster community health and resilience.

Resilience, argue behavioral and social scientists Joie D. Acosta and Elka Gotfryd, should not be viewed as a goal in and of itself, nor as an outcome of a plan or its implementation. Rather, they say, it is a characteristic of a community that is well connected and therefore responsive to challenges as they arise in real time.

Communities cannot be expected to overcome the acute stress associated with a disaster if they are not prepared to cope with day-to-day stress in healthy ways.—Joie D. Acosta

Through this lens, Acosta and Gotfryd do not want practitioners and theorists to ask, "How do we build resilient communities?" but rather, "How can we best nurture the capacity of our communities to organize and respond to stress in healthy ways?" More specific questions flow from there: What kinds of governance structures can support individual and communal quotidian stability in the face of impending economic and environmental challenges? How can we shift from reactive policies and plans to proactive ones?

To find answers, Acosta and Gotfryd look to what they call "regenerative principles of systemic health" as a framework for designing more effective models of governance. Fueled by mutually beneficial, collaborative relationships, these models work in place of existing systems that force groups to compete for resources in a zero-sum game.

Joie D. Acosta and Elka Gotfryd, *Spotlight: Social Infrastructure as a Pathway to Resilience* In: *Community Resilience*. Edited by: Alonzo L. Plough, Oxford University Press (2021). © Robert Wood Johnson Foundation.
DOI: 10.1093/oso/9780197559383.003.0014

In a workshop presented by Acosta and Gotfryd at the 2019 Sharing Knowledge conference in Houston, participants took part in a scenario-based, role-playing game designed to delve into these regenerative principles and to explore their potential applications to governance and planning. In groups of 10, nearly 50 participants acted as members of the Anytown Resilience Plan Committee, an advisory committee organized by the mayor of the fictitious city of Anytown, U.S.A.

With a population of 75,000, Anytown shares a story with many small American cities: Situated along the Sumkinda River, Anytown relies heavily on the local steel manufacturing company for employment and a consistent tax base. It is home to a low-income, predominantly Black community to the south and an affluent, predominantly White community to the north. Students and tourists come to admire Anytown's Gothic Revival architecture, although many of the historic buildings are dilapidated and condemned. Given the increased storm intensity and rising water levels in recent years, the Anytown municipal government predicts that its levee will become ineffective in preventing storm-induced flooding. A recent bout of torrential rain prompted the mayor to convene the advisory committee.

To start the workshop, each group was given the same set of 10 characters to play—including the mayor, the chief of police, the college dean, the YMCA outreach coordinator, and a number of municipal department heads—in order to highlight common dynamics among government officials, community organizations, and others with a role in decision-making and planning. By having all of the groups engage with the same content, Acosta and Gotfryd predicted that they would unearth some of the same systemic barriers to resilience as well as others that reflect unique group dynamics and personalities. For example, most groups soon identified racial tensions as a primary barrier to resilience, noting that an antiracism lens needs to be focused on any plan or policy. Another common barrier, the groups agreed, is that governments tend to focus on short-term rather than long-term gains.

Findings surfaced by this exercise were in line with Gotfryd and Acosta's theoretical framework: Noncollaborative and siloed structures of governance create conditions in which plans and policies are limited to focusing on "disaster preparedness" rather than "community resilience." In other words, preparedness plans are typically short term, disaster centered, and narrowly defined by government agencies; plans that focus on resilience are long-term, ongoing efforts to build and nurture everyday relationships that are crucial to responding to both chronic stressors (e.g., economic stress and social rifts) and acute stressors (e.g., natural disasters).

As the workshop drew to a close, it was apparent that this message had been embraced. One participant expressed an objection to focusing on resilience as a goal, noting that "communities are resilient because they have to be, not because they choose to be." Gotfryd agreed, concluding with this summation:

"We are not working toward resilience. We are building responsive social infrastructure. And when communities have responsive social infrastructure in place, they are naturally more resilient. That's the goal."

Houston Comes Together After Hurricane Harvey

Julie B. Kaplow, PhD, ABPP, Director, Trauma and Grief Center at the Hackett Center for Mental Health

Bakeyah S. Nelson, PhD, MA, Executive Director, Air Alliance Houston

Umair A. Shah, MD, MPH, Executive Director, Harris County Public Health

Renee Wizig-Barrios, Senior Vice President, Chief Philanthropy Officer, Greater Houston Community Foundation

In the face of environmental threats exacerbated by climate change and human behavior, perhaps no community better illustrates the perpetual commitment required to sustain resilience than the largest one in the Lone Star State—Harris County, which is home to the state's largest city, Houston.

For nearly two decades, Houston and Harris County, which surrounds the city, have been tested by forces that have demanded almost constant recovery efforts. A wide range of events, from petrochemical gas explosions and hurricanes to disease outbreaks and flooding, has resulted in what Umair A. Shah, executive director of Harris County Public Health (HCPH), describes as a continual process of preparing for, enduring, and moving forward after devastation. As chapter 10: "Strengthening the Response to Disasters and Trauma" amply demonstrated, strategies to foster resilience in the face of these events are essential.

Resilience is not just recovering after an emergency. Resilience is how a community can grow stronger than it was prior to the emergency. That's why, after disasters, you often see mottos like "Boston Strong or Houston Strong;" resilient

Julie B. Kaplow, Bakeyah S. Nelson, Umair A. Shah, and Renee Wizig-Barrios, *Houston Comes Together After Hurricane Harvey* In: *Community Resilience*. Edited by: Alonzo L. Plough, Oxford University Press (2021). © Robert Wood Johnson Foundation. DOI: 10.1093/oso/9780197559383.003.0015 *communities want to be defined by the strength shown after a disaster, and not the disaster itself.*—Umair A. Shah

This chapter explores the postdisaster impacts of Hurricane Harvey and the continuing efforts to recover since the storm hit on August 26, 2017. Shah describes the dynamics of a diverse county and the public health response to Hurricane Harvey's devastation. Julie B. Kaplow of Texas Children's Hospital's Trauma and Grief Center highlights the extensive outreach and services that have been developed for children, emphasizing the unique needs of young people whose lives are shaped by disasters. Bakeyah S. Nelson of Air Alliance Houston explains why Houston serves as a cautionary tale for what can happen when natural disasters and human-driven environmental disasters collide. And in "Spotlight: Helping Those Who Need It Most," Renee Wizig-Barrios describes how the Greater Houston Community Foundation, supported by an outpouring of contributions after the storm, put a priority on helping at-risk populations.

By highlighting the region's resilience efforts, this chapter suggests the questions that loom large as the impacts of climate change accelerate: Can the Houston/Harris County experience serve as a model for how other communities can move forward after disasters? Or is it a lesson in the limits of a community's ability to adapt?[1]

"We Are Still Recovering"

Harris County is the most populous county in Texas and the third largest county in the nation, with 4.8 million people spread out over 1,778 square miles in the southeastern corner of the state, making it bigger than Rhode Island.[2] Houston, the county seat, claims 2.3 million of these residents within its boundaries, which makes it the largest city in Texas and the fourth largest city in the United States.[3] Shah notes that residents speak over 145 languages, and that Harris County is 43 percent Hispanic or Latino, 29 percent White, 18 percent Black, and about 7 percent Asian.[4]

"We are big, we are diverse, we are complex," says Shah. "It has so many positives for us, but it's also then a challenge to serve those health needs and incorporate those cultural perspectives."

Harvey: An Unprecedented Storm That's Also Familiar

Shah, who is fond of the archetypal myth that "everything is bigger in Texas," is also the first to admit that "unfortunately, so are our challenges."

When Hurricane Harvey made landfall just south of Houston, the National Weather Service had already issued a dire warning: "This event is unprecedented, and all impacts are unknown and beyond anything experienced." The storm stalled over Harris County, dumping 14 months' worth of rainfall in four days throughout the area, breaking the record for the most rainfall from a single storm in the United States. When the rain stopped, nearly one-third of the county was under water from a hurricane that ultimately caused $125 billion in flood damage; destroyed or damaged 135,000 homes; impacted 13 million residents and killed 68 people. It was the deadliest hurricane in Texas in nearly 100 years.

While Harvey was unprecedented in many ways, the devastation it caused was tragically familiar. As the *New York Times* reported, these "disasters aren't just becoming more severe but also more frequent,"[5] and the inequitable and increasingly onerous impact of climate change on low-income communities and communities of color played out in the Houston area. (See chapter 12: "The Environmental Justice Imperative.")

Public health emergencies are nothing new to Harris County, which faced some two dozen of them from 2001 to 2019. A list curated by Shah includes viral threats like measles and Zika; chemical explosions linked to the region's petrochemical industry; and storms that included not only direct hits like Hurricanes Harvey, Ike, and Allison, but also Katrina and others that hit hardest elsewhere but led thousands of evacuees to pour in. "We are a community that has been impacted probably more than any other community in the country on a repeated basis," Shah notes.

Public Health: The Offensive Line in Community Well-Being

A former emergency department physician who has led HCPH since 2013, Shah routinely uses a sports metaphor to describe the work of public health. "Building healthy communities is what public health is all about. We are like the offensive line of a football team. Everyone thinks of doctors and hospitals when it comes to good health, just like everybody thinks of the quarterback in football. But it's public health—the offensive line—that's doing everything it can behind the scenes to ensure the health, well-being, and resilience of our community. The difference is that, in football, we keep investing in the offensive line if you have a winning season. In public health, we do the opposite. When public health is successful, we 'gut' the offensive line. Look at measles rates or tuberculosis. Things get better and we decide that public health is no longer needed. This under-investment in public health remains a big problem."

The deeply held values of the Harris County Public Health Department, notes Alonzo Plough, PhD, chief science officer at the Robert Wood Johnson Foundation (RWJF), inspired the conference theme: "Community Resilience: Innovation, Engagement, and Equity." HCPH officials respond to a wide range of concerns, including but not limited to assessing health challenges after hurricanes and chemical explosions; providing dental services, vaccinations, and other clinical services at health and wellness facilities; monitoring water and food safety at businesses and homes; reducing drug abuse, youth vaping, and neighborhood nuisances; controlling mosquitoes and rescuing animals; and conducting health screenings.

Shah is particularly proud of several initiatives that the department embraced after Hurricane Harvey:

- **Mobile Health Village:** The county has eight mobile units—called a Mobile Health Village—that provide a range of health and well-being services to the community. After the storm, they all traveled throughout the county. "We essentially took the entirety of our programming and put it on wheels," says Shah. "We said, 'Ok, community, we know you're not mobile, but right down the street from you we have a Mobile Health Village that you can come to and get vaccinations for your children or your dog, learn about mosquito prevention and environmental cleanup, take a mental health break.' This really goes to the heart of our cornerstone values."
- **"The Health App That Beat Hurricane Harvey"**[6]**:** During and after the storm, health officials used video directly observed therapy (vDOT) to monitor tuberculosis patients who must take daily medications, often for an extended period of time. Only two of the 61 vDOT patients in Harris County missed their doses of medication during this difficult time, while those patients not on vDOT missed doses and saw their course of therapy extended. This app gained national prominence after Harvey for its success.
- **CASPER:** The health department conducted four hurricane-related surveys called CASPER—Community Assessment for Public Health Emergency Responses. In what Shah calls a remarkable effort, public health staff spent days going door to door within weeks of Hurricane Harvey, and then returned in September 2018 and February 2019 to better understand the recovery needs still present in the communities affected by the storm. These data were compiled and then used for preparedness planning and response activities.

"It's easy to count people in our health care system, but how do you get good data when people are cleaning up their homes or their vehicles and putting their lives back together?" asks Shah. "We were literally going into the community and doing primary data collection to understand how we could better serve our community."

CASPER surveyors often encountered deeply unsettling situations. After the hurricane, teams that visited northwest Harris County, which had been essentially cut off from all services, "came back tearful, really shaken," recalls Shah. The message staff got from angry residents was, "Let me tell you what you all have not done."

> *Residents were not just angry, but at times, aggravated with our teams. They were so frustrated with government, with media, with the way people were portraying that things were getting better when things were not getting better for them.*—Umair A. Shah

- **The Texas Flood Registry**[7]: In conjunction with Rice University and other partners, the health department helped implement a Hurricane Harvey Registry, now known as the Texas Flood Registry, to develop a chronological, prospective snapshot of what happened in the community from the moment Hurricane Harvey landed. The intent was to better understand the health, housing, and environmental impacts of such a major storm. "Not six months later, but in the midst of the storm, we have information about what residents are experiencing and how they are recovering," says Shah. "The registry informs policy, services, and, really, at the end of the day, it continues to keep us honest about what people are going through."
- **Enhanced communications through videos:** In the days and weeks following Hurricane Harvey, Shah and a team of public health employees ventured into neighborhoods to videotape what they saw, an effort not only to document the devastation but also to record the despair of the experience and the faces of resilience. Since September 2017, the public health team has revisited these individuals several times, producing more than 40 videos, many still accessible online and still just as raw, emotional, and powerful as the day they were made.[8] Shah and his team adopted a phrase from epidemiologist Sir Austin Bradford Hill to describe what he saw—and will never forget:

> *Statistics are truly human beings with the tears wiped off.*—Sir Austin Bradford Hill

Behind the Statistics, People and Their Words of Resilience

Nearly four years have passed since Hurricane Harvey made landfall in Texas, but Shah can still repeat verbatim some of his videotaped conversations during the months that followed.

There was a woman named Xiomi with brown hair and sad eyes, who had to evacuate to a local hotel when her house flooded, only to bolt awake at the sound of the hotel's air conditioning turning on. As the water hit the "drip pan" under the unit—*drip, drip, dripping* into the pan—she began to have flashbacks of the rising water in her home. "Even today, I have nightmares. But. I. Am. Better," she said, her eyes tearing up, her voice heavy with emotion born of the continuing struggle behind her words. "My house—it is back together. But how are we going to get back to our *life*?"[9]

Then there was Eddie, an unlikely Pittsburgh Steelers fan in Houston who stayed with his extended family on the second floor of his flooded home for four-and-a-half months, working to rebuild a house that ultimately could not be saved. "This family had to come together. One of the reasons we left, my grandson was nine, and we didn't want to traumatize him anymore," said Eddie, his voice calm but resigned. "How do you process all of this, knowing that Mother Nature is not kind? Constantly, it's on your mind."[10]

And there were David and Bertha, who lost their home, as did everyone else on their waterlogged block, their friendly street turned into mounds of debris. "We had six feet of water inside the house, it was completely destroyed, it was very sad. It was bad," said David. "But we don't dwell on the negative. Whatever comes our way, just keep going." Added Bertha, "We're still working on this house. And we're still working on our life."[11]

These stories, Shah argues, reflect an aspect of storm-related recovery that gets lost after the television news vans and media reporters move on, but they are a reality that public health professionals and impacted communities face every day. The road to recovery is not a sprint, it is a marathon. And those with fewer resources and markedly less support take longer to bounce back.

> *The headlines have gone away. But our communities are still recovering. It's going to take a long time.*—Umair A. Shah

Children Are Traumatized Long After the Storm

In August 2017, Julie B. Kaplow was named director of the Trauma and Grief Center at Texas Children's Hospital, a center that she had originally established in 2012 at the University of Michigan and then expanded when she moved to Texas. Kaplow brought with her an expertise in childhood bereavement and grief that stemmed from her undergraduate and PhD studies in clinical psychology and childhood trauma. As a student and scholar, she was struck by the fact that many children who had lost a parent were able to adjust, while others got stuck. "I was very interested in what helped some children who had experienced objectively horrific events do well over time, while others could not move forward," she says.

Less than one month after her appointment, Kaplow, who had never lived through a hurricane before, confronted a special cohort of traumatized children: those who survived Hurricane Harvey.

Hurricane-Exposed Youth and Tools for Resilience

A wealth of existing studies shows that experiencing a hurricane and being exposed to extensive flooding place youth at risk for post-traumatic stress disorder; depression; anxiety; and in some cases that involve loss of life, persistent complex bereavement disorder.[12]

Kaplow also knew that bereavement is the most common form of trauma, and the most disruptive for children.[13] Says Kaplow, "One of our recent studies showed that of 14,000 students across the U.S., sudden bereavement was actually the strongest predictor of school failure, above and beyond any other form of trauma, including sexual abuse, physical abuse, or exposure to violence."

One of 100 sites in the National Child Traumatic Stress Network—which was created by Congress in 2000 to raise awareness and increase services to children who experience or witness traumatic events—the Trauma and Grief Center already specialized in bereavement and the interplay of trauma and grief. In the aftermath of Harvey, Kaplow knew that "we needed all hands on deck to deploy our trauma and grief clinicians wherever they were needed." She highlights three key resources:

- **Mental health services:** The Trauma and Grief Center partnered with Mental Health America to provide mental health services to students and training for school-based clinicians and counselors in some of the hardest-hit schools and communities across Harris County. In schools where counselors were trained in intervention strategies, notes Kaplow, "We are seeing reductions in post-traumatic stress disorder, maladaptive grief, and depression." In addition to providing training, Kaplow used funding support from the Hurricane Harvey Relief Fund to deploy trauma and grief clinicians to outpatient clinics in high-risk areas, ensuring that families and children receive not only medical care but also mental health care services. (For more about the Relief Fund, and the projects it funded through the Greater Houston Community Foundation, see "Spotlight: Helping Those Who Need It Most" at the end of this chapter.)
- **Mobile mental health units:** Supported by grants from RWJF and the Center for Disaster Philanthropy, the center expanded its mobile mental

health services after the hurricane. Trauma and grief specialists now travel to five hard-hit schools that also have the highest levels of immigrant youth.[14]

Using the mobile units to serve undocumented youth, says Kaplow, serves two purposes: addressing a high-need population and correcting a significant health disparity. "Not only have they experienced traumas before coming to this country—which is why they were fleeing—but as soon as they get here they're impacted by the floods and the hurricane. So this is a very, very important group that has often been overlooked. We recognize that most of our underserved and especially our immigrant families would either have difficulty traveling to the hospital or would not feel comfortable coming to the hospital."

- **HEART (Hurricane Exposure, Adversity, and Recovery Tool)— Assessing Youth Exposed to Hurricanes:** When Kaplow discovered that most post-hurricane risk-screening and assessment tools were designed primarily for adults, she knew she had to create a new one for children that used "child-friendly" language and was culturally appropriate. Such tools are critically important to identify youth who have been exposed to potent hurricane-related risk factors, who are most at risk for post-traumatic stress, and help allocate resources and mental health services.[15]

Through the Trauma and Grief Center, Kaplow helped launch the Harvey Resilience and Recovery Program, targeted at children and families.[16] Within this program, she and her team created HEART, adapting it from an earlier assessment tool created by the National Child Traumatic Stress Network. HEART uses 29 statements, specifically designed for children and adolescents, that require yes/no answers in order to uncover risk factors that predict post-traumatic stress disorders.[17] Among the statements are the following:

> I got hurt. . . . Someone in my family or a close friend died. . . . My pet got badly hurt and died. . . . I had to leave my house very quickly. . . . I was trapped in my house. . . . Someone rescued me. . . . My family was afraid to ask for help because we thought we might get in trouble. . . . I had to move out of my house. . . . I had to go to a new school. . . . My family is having a hard time. . . . I was in another disaster.—HEART statements to which children gave yes/no answers

The HEART tool (along with another measure of child post-traumatic stress symptoms called the UCLA PTSD Reaction Index, Brief Form[18]) helped Kaplow and her team discover a grim statistic: Children who appeared least resilient after Harvey and who identified as having post-traumatic stress disorder were those who had experienced prior losses and trauma. This information offered insights into Kaplow's early career question about why some people bounce back from adversity and others do not. The team also kept hearing from teachers and parents that Harvey actually had a silver lining of sorts: By focusing attention on pre-existing mental health suffering, it allowed Houston's traumatized children to finally receive treatment for issues that had never been adequately addressed.

Kaplow plans to create a Disaster Response Team specifically to respond to trauma and crises throughout the region. "Because it's not just the hurricane. It's the Santa Fe High School shooting, the Odessa shooting, the El Paso shooting, separation and immigration issues, the high rates of suicide. That weighs heavily on me," she says, adding after a long pause, "We're essentially needed everywhere."

Emphasizing that treating traumatized children requires a long-term effort, Kaplow notes that stress and bereavement-related disorders tend to be most acute six to eight months following a traumatic event and may not emerge for up to 18 months later. "Children are still showing up" two years after Hurricane Harvey, she says. And mental health experts now report that the constant threat of natural disasters in the Houston area has made some children "hypervigilant" and more prone to anxiety.

The minute it starts to rain, there is an almost immediate panic that takes over in many children. "Oh God, are we going to flood again?"—Julie B. Kaplow

Air Pollution in Houston: A Second STORM

The fear that Houston children experience during a rainfall is part of an ominous cloud—both metaphorically and literally—that hangs over the entire Houston region. When it comes to air quality in Houston, Bakeyah S. Nelson of Air Alliance Houston described a desperate situation that is a daily norm but worsened significantly immediately after Hurricane Harvey.

The backdrop is that the Houston region is home to some 400 types of hazardous facilities—ranging from waste dumps to chemical plants and including two of the four largest oil refineries in the country. Harris County has been called "the center of the largest petrochemical complex in the Western Hemisphere," and more than 1.7 million county residents live within half a mile of the region's nearly 10,000 miles of pipeline.[19] And Houston's pollution-producing industries, chemical facilities, and warehouses filled with hazardous materials are widely scattered, which means the damage can be widely dispersed as well.[20]

According to Nelson, these hazardous facilities and oil operations release be-tween five and six million pounds of illegal pollution into the region every year.[21] (Illegal pollution exceeds the air emissions allowed by permit and must be re-ported to the state.)

When Hurricane Harvey hit the Houston area, the storm "knocked down smokestacks, damaged pipelines, broke chemical storage tanks, and flooded hazardous waste sites, causing poisonous runoff to spill," the *Houston Chronicle* reported.[22] As facilities were compromised, they released nearly eight million pounds of air pollution before, during, and after the storm.

> *We had a year's worth of pollution in just a matter of weeks. It was a second storm of pollution.*—Bakeyah S. Nelson

Navigating Air Quality Post-Harvey

Nelson is the first to admit that "we did not have a good handle on what people and the communities were going through" in terms of air quality. She notes that up to 75 percent of the area's stationary air monitoring network had been turned off and secured by the state ahead of Harvey's landfall—a time when many oil refineries and other facilities were shutting down, resulting in the emission of ex-cess pollution that one newspaper described as "millions of pounds of hazardous air pollution." And they spewed out even more when they restarted.[23]

When Nelson learned that almost no air monitoring was taking place, Air Alliance Houston began working with the Environmental Defense Fund to se-cure a mobile air monitoring unit to gather air samples. Their target was areas where industries were already reporting elevated emissions levels to the state and where residents were calling to complain about chemical odors in their neighborhoods.[24] Desperate to help, Nelson and others tried to collect air samples themselves and promptly got sick. At one point, the mobile air monitoring unit detected a benzene plume, not visible to the human eye, over one of the most vulnerable communities in southeastern Houston. Known as Manchester, it is in close proximity to the Houston Ship Channel, which is dotted by many chemical plants, refineries, and sewage facilities. The amount of benzene, a widely known human carcinogen, was significantly higher than health-protective guidelines set by other states, and Nelson remembers that officials "considered evacuating the community."[25]

Information that verified the depths of this colossal air monitoring failure during and after Hurricane Harvey continued to emerge well into 2019 through investigations, Congressional testimony, and special reports.

- A year after the storm, a probe by the *Houston Chronicle* and the Associated Press found that the environmental damage caused by Harvey was "much bigger than authorities reported. Benzene, vinyl chloride, butadiene, and other known human carcinogens were among the dozens of tons of industrial chemicals released throughout Houston's petrochemical corridor and surrounding neighborhoods and waterways following Harvey's torrential rains."[26]

- In a scathing opinion piece published in the *Houston Chronicle* in September 2018, Nelson wrote that Houston had fallen further behind than ever in fighting air pollution: In 2018 alone, companies in Harris County reported more than 150 pollution releases that exceeded their state permits, actions that went largely unpunished by the Environmental Protection Agency (EPA). From 2011 to 2016, virtually all (at least 97 percent) of illegal releases occurred without penalty.[27]

- In February 2019, Nelson testified at a congressional hearing that low levels of enforcement by the EPA and the Texas Commission on Environmental Quality (TCEQ) are "endangering the health of local communities in Houston. Years ago, the EPA had recognized the need to make preventing chemical disasters a national enforcement initiative, but communities in Houston haven't seen EPA make good on that promise. . . . The agency is instead turning its back on communities that need enforcement the most."

- In news that shocked nearly everyone, the *Los Angeles Times* disclosed for the first time in March 2019 that the air monitoring situation was so dire in Houston after Harvey that highly trained NASA officials had reached out to offer sophisticated systems and expertise to help monitor air pollution after the hurricane—and that the EPA and TCEQ had turned NASA's offer down, basically saying, "No, thank you." Such a negligent response, which is now under investigation by Congress,[28] was an unforgiveable mistake, Nelson believes.

"The TCEQ and EPA have failed every single person in our region, but particularly communities of color and low wealth that live closest to the facilities that were damaged and caused millions of pounds of harmful air pollution to be released during Harvey," Nelson wrote when news of the NASA offer first surfaced. "This decision is yet another tragic example of these agencies failing to prioritize people over industry and continuing the legacy of environmental injustice. These decisions fuel the production of health inequities and contribute to the vast differences in life expectancy between communities in the Houston region."[29]

*Houston and Hurricane Harvey serve as a cautionary tale for what it's like
to have this high a concentration of hazardous facilities.*—Bakeyah S. Nelson

Lessons Learned

For Nelson, the complete failure of the air monitoring system during Hurricane
Harvey underscored the urgency of avoiding a similar situation in the future.
Among the essential steps she believes are needed:

- **A backup air quality monitoring plan must be in place if an existing one
  malfunctions or is shut down.** Post-Harvey, Nelson says that Houston and
  Harris County began to develop a low-cost, mobile air monitoring network
  for the region. At a minimum, a disaster-based air quality monitoring plan
  should be developed to monitor the air near communities that are closest to
  toxic facilities. Likewise, facilities in closest proximity to residents should be
  held to a higher monitoring standard.
- **A multi-issue policy agenda is needed to better coordinate advocacy
  efforts at the intersection of pollution, place, and public health.** Post-
  Harvey, Nelson and Jennifer Powis of the Powis Firm formed the Coalition
  for Environment, Equity, and Resilience (CEER)—a group of over 25 organizations representing environmental, social justice, transportation, affordable
  housing, and other community groups. Through a multidisciplinary policy
  agenda that guides its advocacy efforts, and under the leadership of its new
  director, Iris Gonzalez, CEER is now working on several initiatives that aim
  to strengthen Houston's ability to rebound equitably from disasters in the future; minimize the kinds of public health risks that communities faced during
  Harvey; and hold leaders accountable for environmental disasters that can no
  longer be excused as what Nelson calls the "price of economic prosperity" in
  Houston.[30]
- **Federal and state agencies should establish safety threshold levels for air
  pollutants.** "In the situation like Manchester," explains Nelson, "no one really knew what to do because there was no framework in place that said, 'After
  benzene hits a certain level, then residents should be evacuated.' That framework should be in place." Adopting air quality thresholds during disasters can
  help to inform decision-making about when to evacuate residents, enhance
  public awareness, and reduce potential public health impacts.
- **Better communication must be established.** Nelson notes that communication about air quality concerns among city, county, state, and federal
  agencies during the storm had been inconsistent, although by late 2019 communication channels between city and county officials had improved. She
  also emphasized the need for a toxic alert system to provide timely warnings

to communities when a chemical incident occurs. And communities deserve to be engaged before environmental emergencies "so they are not always having to react to situations that emerge using information that is either inaccurate and/or not timely," she adds.

A Final Word

In mid-September 2019, Tropical Depression Imelda unexpectedly pummeled parts of Texas with so much rain that Governor Greg Abbott declared a state of disaster in 13 counties, including Harris County. On September 19, two years and two weeks after Hurricane Harvey, a newspaper headline captured the experience: "For Some in Texas, Imelda's Heavy Rain Feels Like Harvey 2.0."[31]

Renee Wizig-Barrios of the Greater Houston Community Foundation notes that the foundation was particularly attuned to the needs of undocumented individuals after Imelda, and that services were already in place to help those who were most vulnerable.

Nelson admits that at times she and her staff suffer from "resilience burnout." She now views Houston's response to repeated storms as both a tremendous opportunity—"We can show the rest of the country that we can step up and do things differently"—and a reminder that decision-makers are still pursuing "this path that's almost self-destructive. It's very difficult to reconcile the two. It's like you're in the midst of a community that knows how to come together in the face of a crisis, but as soon as that emergency is over, it is back to business as usual."

Nelson wrestles all the time with whether to remain in Houston—or take her family and flee the place she has called home since 2006. "On the one hand, I want to stay and do all that I can to help. But on the other hand, having the level of information that I have about the threats that exist here, is it irresponsible to continue to live here?"

Kaplow is more optimistic. She believes that "we were more prepared for Imelda because we had gone through Harvey. I absolutely think of Houston as a resilient community."

Shah, perhaps, spoke for everyone who lives with the reality that the next storm, the next environmental emergency, the next health epidemic is inevitable. His next words, spoken before the Covid-19 pandemic, were prescient. "Our work," he concludes, "is never done."

I think that's really the story of our community. We sort of get beaten down but we get right back up. And we are even stronger in how we then face the next emergency that comes our way. Because, in our community, no doubt it will.—Umair A. Shah

Spotlight

Helping Those Who Need It Most

Renee Wizig-Barrios, Senior Vice President, Chief Philanthropy Officer, Greater Houston Community Foundation

After more than 20 years of experience in disaster relief philanthropy, the staff at Greater Houston Community Foundation knew the world was watching when Hurricane Harvey devastated communities in Houston and Harris County. With the level of media attention before and after the storm made landfall, the foundation anticipated a generous response, but not of the magnitude that actually materialized.

Through donations from all over the world, the Hurricane Harvey Relief Fund raised more than $114 million from 127,000 unique donors in the year after the storm, making it the largest fund in the foundation's history. Donations came in equal measure from individuals, foundations, and corporations. The fund also made history because of its origin story—City and county government forces together approached the foundation about launching the relief effort for Houston and Harris County.

Though Harvey hit all communities and people of all income levels, the poorest areas bore the brunt of the crisis, as they so often do. Recovery operations were slower there, and those who needed the social service system most found it extremely difficult to navigate. The Relief Fund Advisory Board decided to focus its efforts largely on economically disadvantaged and at-risk populations—low-income, disabled, elderly and medically fragile people, veterans, and undocumented immigrants. Recognizing that "FEMA [Federal Emergency Management Agency] would not be helping the undocumented in our community," as the foundation's Renee Wizig-Barrios points out, both Houston and Harris County were adamant that philanthropy needed to reach out to immigrant families. (For more about the special challenges immigrant families faced in the wake of the storm, see chapter 4: "Immigrants in America: Stories of Trauma and Resilience.")

Renee Wizig-Barrios, *Spotlight: Helping Those Who Need It Most* In: *Community Resilience*. Edited by: Alonzo L. Plough, Oxford University Press (2021). © Robert Wood Johnson Foundation. DOI: 10.1093/oso/9780197559383.003.0016

"We had some push back—because this was an equal-opportunity storm," she says. "But we talk a lot about equity and we knew, based on data, that it would be harder for people to recover who didn't have insurance, who were otherwise marginalized, who didn't have savings, who were undocumented, who couldn't access family members who could help them."

The Hurricane Harvey Relief Fund conducted five rounds of funding, benefiting almost 440,000 people in some 158,000 households, by July 2019. Grants were primarily allocated in these categories: $42 million for home repair and temporary housing; $14.6 million for case management to navigate the recovery system; $15 million for direct financial assistance (e.g., emergency funds to pay rent, buy food, fix cars); $7 million for furnishings; $6 million for behavioral health care services; $5 million for basic needs requests; and $3 million for legal services, particularly around issues of equity and fairness that often involved FEMA appeals, title clearances, landlord disputes, or filing insurance forms. The funded services were available through July 2020.

Highlights of these projects include the following:

- **Harvey Home Connect:** Established to help those who needed home repair services, Harvey Home Connect was a veritable one-stop, home repair clearinghouse. Case managers helped process applications and matched homeowners to professionals who then assessed the damage and connected owners to vetted home repair agencies and contractors. By July 2019, the project had repaired 633 homes; assessments or repairs of another 425 homes were in process. Wizig-Barrios noted that much of the work done through Harvey Home Connect was underway long before home repair dollars from FEMA finally began to be dispersed in June 2019.

- **Northwest Assistance Ministries (NAM):** Rosewood Mobile Home Community was in dire need of recovery assistance when NAM set out to determine eligibility for relief services. In one day, 74 staff members and volunteers conducted 55 comprehensive assessments, work that might more typically have taken three to four months. By July 2019, seven trailers had been replaced and 12 trailers had been repaired, with dedicated community members joining the repair effort.

- **Mental health impacts of Hurricane Harvey:** Supported by a $2.1 million grant from the relief fund, the Texas Children's Hospital and Mental Health America partnered to provide mental health services to approximately 247,000 students in some of the hardest hit schools and communities across Harris County.

The spirit of collaboration that inspired the Hurricane Harvey Relief Fund and led to its focus on equitable philanthropy remains inspirational to the broader philanthropic community. "While the troubling memories [of Hurricane Harvey] are in our history and in our hearts, we also remember the hope, the heroes, and the overwhelming spirit of togetherness Houstonians displayed through it all," the organizers noted in the fund's two-year update. "We remember neighbors helping neighbors, strangers helping strangers, and most of all, we remember the strength and resilience of our community in the face of disaster."

The Environmental Justice Imperative

Patrick N. Breysse, PhD, National Center for Environmental Health/Agency for Toxic Substances and Disease Registry, Centers for Disease Control and Prevention

Robert Bullard, PhD, Distinguished Professor, Dean, Barbara Jordan-Mickey Leland School of Public Affairs, Texas Southern University

Elizabeth Sawin, PhD, Co-Founder and Co-Director, Climate Interactive

Beverly Wright, PhD, Founding Executive Director, Deep South Center for Environmental Justice

As the hottest decade on record came to a close in 2019, the impacts of climate change were projected to increase over the next century, triggering everything from rising and warmer seas, weather-related disasters, increasingly erratic temperatures, and more illness and disease.[1] These widely studied and well-documented consequences will impact low-income communities and communities of color hardest, putting them in harm's way more frequently and severely limiting their ability to recover.[2]

"The people at greatest risk of serious harm from these climate change-related events include children, the elderly, people with chronic health conditions, the economically-marginalized and communities of color," says Robert Wood Johnson Foundation's (RWJF's) Alonzo Plough. "Those who are already vulnerable stand to be most affected."[3]

While the preceding chapters in this part focused on the need for resilience in the face of acute and chronic stressors of all kinds, each of them also landed on climate change as one of the most significant drivers of that stress.

In this chapter, contributors probe the interface of climate change and human health, with an emphasis on underserved communities. Patrick N. Breysse of the

Patrick N. Breysse, Robert Bullard, Elizabeth Sawin, and Beverly Wright, *The Environmental Justice Imperative*
In: *Community Resilience*. Edited by: Alonzo L. Plough, Oxford University Press (2021). © Robert Wood Johnson Foundation.
DOI: 10.1093/oso/9780197559383.003.0017

Centers for Disease Control and Prevention (CDC) reviews the health effects of climate change and describes how the CDC's Climate and Health Program helps bolster local, state, tribal, and territorial efforts to protect vulnerable communities. Robert Bullard of Texas Southern University and Beverly Wright of the Deep South Center for Environmental Justice confront the racial inequity of climate change and chemical disasters. Bullard channels the legacy of slavery as he demonstrates how states that once enslaved people now house the communities hit hardest by climate change.[4] Through her work with the Deep South Center for Environmental Justice, Wright describes the unique ways that local communities confront the negative impacts of climate change. And in a Spotlight, Climate Interactive's Elizabeth Sawin presents a concept called "multisolving" that addresses climate change solutions that also have health benefits.

> Climate change doesn't just harm our health. It deepens inequities.—RWJF, Health and Climate Solutions program[5]

Inequitable Health Effects

Patrick N. Breysse, who leads the CDC's efforts to investigate the relationship between environmental factors and health, captures the bottom line in one simple sentence. "When seas and temperatures rise," he says, "health consequences are not equal."

With information and charts from the CDC's Climate and Health Program—established 10 years ago to help public health agencies prepare[6]—Breysse laid out three interrelated pathways for the harms of climate change: It can affect health directly, spread diseases, and disrupt mental health and well-being.

> If you look across these categories, we see a pretty constant pattern in terms of what it means to be vulnerable to climate change.—Patrick N. Breysse

Climate Change Affects Health Directly

The consequences of extreme weather, extreme heat, and air pollution have direct effects on health, explains Breysse.

- **Extreme weather**—characterized by increased frequency and severity of heavy downpours, floods, droughts, and major storms—can lead to injury, illness, displacement, and death. Extreme weather can also trigger more air pollution, leading to greater risks of asthma and cardiovascular disease and a surge in vector-borne diseases.

The Fourth National Climate Assessment, produced by the U.S. Global Change Research Program in 2018, concluded, "People who are already vulnerable, including lower-income and marginalized communities, have lower capacity to prepare for and cope with extreme weather and climate-related events and are expected to experience greater impacts."[7]

"This is always front and center when you talk about climate change and health," says Breysse. "The people who are most vulnerable include low-income groups, racial minorities, immigrant groups, Indigenous peoples, children and pregnant women, older adults, persons with disabilities, and persons with pre-existing medical conditions."

- **Extreme heat**—characterized by higher temperatures, increased humidity, and longer and more frequent heat waves—is "probably one of the most important manifestations of climate change on health," says Breysse.

Extreme heat can lead to dehydration, heatstroke, cardiovascular failure and death, while increasing hospitalizations and mortality from a wide variety of diseases. The leading weather-related killer in the United States, extreme heat kills more people every year than tornados, floods, and hurricanes. An estimated 600 to 1,500 heat-related deaths occur in an average summer, and those numbers increase every year.[8] Breysse also notes that these numbers "may be an underestimate, as death records sometimes do not specifically list heat as a contributing cause."

Recent studies showed the inequitable impact of extreme heat:

- o Heat-related deaths among Blacks are 150 to 200 percent more likely than among non-Hispanic Whites, according to a 2008 study by the Environmental Justice and Climate Change initiative.[9]
- o Low-income neighborhoods are hotter than wealthier ones, and poor people bear the brunt of rising heat across the country, according to a 2018 report by National Public Radio (NPR) and the Howard Center for Investigative Journalism at the University of Maryland.[10]
- o Low-income households and communities of color are more likely to live in what's being called urban "heat islands," according to a 2020 journal article published in *Climate*.[11] These heat islands are hotter than the surrounding areas due to an overabundance of concrete and pavements and a lack of green spaces and tree canopies.
- **Air pollution**—characterized by smog, pollen, and also triggered by wildfires—can result in increased asthma morbidity and mortality, allergy attacks, and other respiratory issues, as well as cardiovascular diseases. People with pre-existing conditions are at greatest risk, with an unequal burden again falling on people of color and low-income households.

"I cut my teeth as an environmental health scientist on air pollution research, and one of the most obvious, direct, environmental exposures associated with climate change is an increase in air pollution," says Breysse. "We know that the pollution levels are greatest in the city environments where vulnerable people are often concentrated."

Breysse's assertions are backed by a 2018 Environmental Protection Agency (EPA) report, which found that race, not poverty, was the strongest predictor of exposure to air pollution. Black people face higher exposure to air pollution than Whites, particularly to health-damaging particles linked to burning fossil fuels.[12]

Climate Change Spreads Disease, Disrupts Mental Health

Climate change plays a prominent role in spreading disease through two distinct paths:

- **Contaminated water and food**—caused by higher water temperatures, extreme weather, heavier downpours, rising sea levels, flooding, and humidity—help spread gastrointestinal diseases as well as diseases from bacteria and toxins found in food, drinking water, and swimming areas. As water and food supplies are compromised, malnutrition and diarrheal diseases like cholera and cryptosporidiosis can surface.
- **Insects, ticks, and rodents**—Higher temperatures, changes in rain, and disrupted ecosystems can affect the distribution and spread of insects, ticks, and rodents. These vectors spread diseases like malaria, dengue, hantavirus, Lyme disease, and West Nile virus.

Finally, Breysse argues that climate change can disrupt mental health and well-being. He notes that mental health problems—triggered by increased frequency and severity of extreme weather events—surface as stress, depression, anxiety, post-traumatic stress disorder, and suicidal thoughts.

A recent report by NPR and the University of Maryland's Howard Center was one of the first to document a link between heat and mental health. After analyzing emergency response data from the summer of 2018 in Baltimore, the report found that calls for psychiatric conditions increased by nearly 40 percent when the study's heat index, which factors in heat and humidity to describe how hot the air feels, spiked over 103 degrees.[13]

"This is a poorly investigated aspect of climate change," says Breysse, "but if you don't talk about the mental health dimension, you're not touching on one of the more important parts of the problems."

The CDC's Climate and Health Program

The CDC's Climate and Health Program is designed to bolster local, state, tribal, and territorial efforts to protect their communities. As described by Breysse, the program provides resources for state, local, and tribal health agencies; helps prepare public health practitioners to address the health effects of climate change; and provides community-facing tools, guides, and processes to assess health-related vulnerabilities.

Those efforts are carried out through a framework called Building Resilience Against Climate Effects (BRACE).[14] Working with complex data and projections for future public health concerns, BRACE helps communities determine existing climate health vulnerabilities, project their anticipated health effects, and assess and implement public health interventions. CDC's Climate and Health Program has two main initiatives through which it provides funding and technical assistance:

- **Climate-Ready States and Cities Initiative.** So far, 16 states and two cities have adopted the BRACE framework to pinpoint vulnerabilities and implement adaptation strategies. Here are two examples:
  o To address extreme heat events, the San Francisco Department of Health established a heat vulnerability assessment. In addition to temperature, the assessment includes 22 social and environmental vulnerabilities and identifies factors like heat-absorbing concrete, tree density, older homes without air conditioning, and the presence of older adults, children, and homeless individuals (who are more sensitive to heat). The tool is used by city planners to develop resources, such as parks and tree planting, that increase shade and boost cooling effects.[15,16]
  o The state of Minnesota adopted air quality alert messages to protect individuals from exposure to pollution. Through multiagency collaboration, the climate-related messages target those most sensitive to poor air quality.
- **Climate-Ready Tribes and Territories Initiative.** In partnership with the National Indian Health Board and the Association of State and Territorial Health Officials, the CDC is working with seven tribes to use the BRACE framework to identify climate vulnerabilities and mitigate health impacts. Here are two examples from the initiative, which was phased in from 2016 to 2019:
  o After identifying extreme precipitation, air quality, rising temperatures and humidity, and vector-borne diseases as climate change impacts, the Kaw Nation EPA in Kaw City, Oklahoma, created a series of fact sheets to communicate with their members.[17] The fact sheet "Adverse Health

Effects of Extreme Precipitation," for instance, provides tips on how to avoid food-borne and water-related illnesses.

o After identifying drought, elevated temperatures, storms, flooding, and wildfires as climate change vulnerabilities, the Pala Band of Mission Indians in Pala, California, created extensive information sheets and webinars to describe the problems and their high-risk health impacts, including tips for staying safe during climate-related events.[18]

Poverty and Race

The year 2019 has been called "The Year the World Woke Up to Climate Change." Schoolchildren skipped classes to protest, *Time Magazine* named Swedish teenager and climate activist Greta Thunberg "Person of the Year," protestors took to the streets in cities around the world, and reports from climate scientists and global health organizations grew increasingly dire. "People around the world dragged the climate emergency into the mainstream in 2019," declared *ScienceAlert*, an online news site.[19]

But for environmental justice leaders like Robert Bullard and Beverly Wright, the year simply turned a spotlight on what they have worked tirelessly for decades to share with others: Climate change, together with other natural and human-made health stressors, threatens everyone—with low-income communities and communities of color bearing the brunt of the inequities.[20]

"Though everyone—White, Black, Brown—is now threatened by climate change, the health risks and impacts of climate change are not equally or fairly distributed," says Wright, echoing the CDC's Patrick N. Breysse and the consistent pattern that has been documented throughout this volume.

In the United States, inequities in living and health conditions, as well as political, social and economic power, place low income communities and some communities of color at greater risk for health impacts of climate change.—Beverly Wright

The Father of Environmental Justice: Robert Bullard

Robert Bullard tracks his interest in environmental justice back to the late 1970s when he was a sociology professor at Texas Southern University, teaching a research methods class. During the semester, his wife, attorney Linda McKeever Bullard, asked if he would help collect data for a legal challenge to the location of a municipal landfill in a predominately Black, middle-class community in

Houston. Bullard jumped at the opportunity to engage his students in a real-world study.[21]

After digging into the data, they discovered that all five of the city-owned landfills were located in Black neighborhoods, as were six out of eight city-owned incinerators and three out of four privately owned landfills. That string of findings led Bullard to conclude that 82 percent of all waste dumped in Houston from the 1930s to 1978 had landed in Black neighborhoods. The bias revealed in these findings is especially transparent given that Blacks made up only 25 percent of the Houston population over the four decades studied.[22]

Bullard's research became part of the legal argument in a landmark case called *Bean v. Southwestern Waste Management Corporation*, widely recognized as the first lawsuit to use civil rights law to challenge environmental racism in locating a waste facility. "Of course, we didn't win the case," acknowledges Bullard of the 1979 federal court case that was appealed and finally resolved in 1985. "But we did *win*. We lost the battle but we won the war in terms of launching a research field and expanding that original Houston study to look at what was happening in the South."

We have to understand that the most vulnerable populations in the US and around the world have contributed least to the problem but suffer the pain first, worst, and longest.—Robert Bullard

Statistics and Maps That Don't Lie

Bullard's research not only launched his career as an environmental justice scholar and activist but also inspired his campaign against what he calls "environmental racism."[23] He expanded his initial study on landfill-placement discrimination and went on to write 18 books about related topics. *Dumping in Dixie: Race, Class, and Environmental Quality* was published in 1990; more recently, in 2012, he and Wright co-authored *The Wrong Complexion for Protection*.

At the 2019 *Sharing Knowledge* conference in Houston, Bullard presented a remarkable trove of studies and statistics to illustrate the legacy of environmental racism on health. For instance:

- Blacks are almost three times more likely to die from asthma-related causes, and Black children are four times more likely to be admitted to the hospital for asthma, compared to non-Hispanic White children.[24]
- Regardless of economic status, people of color bear a greater burden from air pollution. Blacks are 79 percent more likely than Whites to live where industrial pollution poses the greatest health danger.[25]

- Citing one of his own books, Bullard notes that in major disasters, the most vulnerable populations generally suffer the earliest and most damaging setbacks because of where they live, their limited income and economic means, and lack of access to health care.[26]
- To illustrate how these disasters widen racial wealth gaps in the United States, Bullard reported on a study showing that White communities gained an average of $126,000 in wealth following the damage and recovery efforts from events like hurricanes and wildfires, while communities of color lose up to $29,000 in personal wealth, on average.[27]

Incorporating a mapping technique similar to ones used by RWJF to chart life expectancy based on zip codes,[28] Bullard demonstrated that areas with a history of poverty, poor health, and past slavery mirror those most impacted by extreme weather events and climate change in the present day. He showed four maps, each highlighted with red blocks of color: slave states and territories in 1860; segregated states in 1950; states with the most people living in poverty in 2010; and states with at least one billion dollars in weather and climate disasters from 1980 to 2012. As he pointed out that all four maps covered a nearly identical swath of the Southeast, Bullard reduced the room to shocked silence.

> Look at that pattern that I'm showing you. Are you getting the picture? Zip code is still one of the most potent predictors of health and well-being, and here's inequality by zip code. You can map that.—Robert Bullard

Tracking Environmental Justice History

Throughout his career, Bullard has attacked environmental racism and worked to expand the environmental justice movement from numerous angles. In 1990, he was part of a group of prominent academics that became known as the Michigan Group, whose work resulted in the creation of the EPA's Work Group on Environmental Equity (later called the Office of Environmental Justice); this is widely acknowledged as the turning point leading the EPA to look at the environment through the lens of race and class.[29] In 1994, when President Bill Clinton signed the first major federal executive order on environmental justice, which required all federal agencies to "make achieving environmental justice part of its mission," Bullard was one of many activists in the Oval Office for the ceremony.[30] In 2019, he was named one of the world's 100 Most Influential People in Climate Policy by Apolitical, a peer-to-peer learning platform for governments.[31]

With over four decades of fighting for environmental justice, Bullard, now a distinguished professor at the same Texas Southern University where he launched his career, is the first to admit that the "quest for environmental justice for all communities has yet to be achieved."[32] But he is not giving up. "Dismantling institutional racism would go a long way in closing environmental health disparities in the United States," he affirms.

It's time for Whites to stop dumping their pollution on people of color.
—Robert Bullard[33]

Mitigating Inequities

Like Bullard, Beverly Wright has made environmental justice her life's work. She steered onto this course after a series of remarkable coincidences completely derailed her original plan to study teenage pregnancy. Consider the following:

Wright's graduate school advisor at the State University of New York at Buffalo was Aldeline Gordon Levine, PhD, the sociologist who wrote the book on Love Canal, a small community located near Niagara Falls that was built on a toxic waste dump and became one of the country's largest environmental pollution disasters.[34] Wright's first academic position at the University of New Orleans put her in the birthplace of the environmental justice movement and the immediate vicinity of "Cancer Alley," an area along the Mississippi River between Baton Rouge and New Orleans distinguished by its proliferation of petrochemical industries and a high rate of cancer in poor communities.

Continuing the pattern, Wright happened to sit next to Robert Bullard at a Southern Sociological Association meeting in the mid-1980s, and he convinced her to collaborate with him on a paper, "The Politics of Pollution: Implications for the Black Community," published in 1986. When Wright later agreed to help Bullard write *Dumping in Dixie,* published in 1990, she knew her days exploring teenage pregnancy were over.

Today, Wright is considered one of the leading members of the environmental justice movement and, like Bullard, was one of the original members of the Michigan Group, helping to launch the EPA's environmental justice efforts. In 1992, she founded the Deep South Center for Environmental Justice, which collaborates with community groups and universities in the American South.[35]

From this platform, Wright continues her work to mitigate the inequities of climate change, focusing especially on children and families harmed by pollution and vulnerable to environmental impacts in the Gulf Coast region. Her commitment reflects Bullard's call to put "equity at the center" of everything.

The Deep South Center for Environmental Justice

For over 28 years, the Deep South Center has worked to bring environmental justice to African-American communities. Its work includes everything from research and education to skills training for men and women that helps them secure jobs in environmental, health, and safety fields. The following are two examples of center-supported programs to mitigate climate change inequities:

- **Gulf Equity Water Corps.** Designed to advance climate justice and raise awareness about sea-level rise and flooding among student leaders in the Gulf Coast region, the corps brings together interns from college and high school settings. They conduct research and receive training on such diverse topics as drainage capacity and flooding in the Lower Ninth Ward in New Orleans to mapping sea-level rise along the Gulf Coast.[36]
- **"Taking Steps Together on Equity & Climate Change: A Report by and for New Orleanians."** This collaborative report, says Wright, "ties together action to achieve equity with action on climate change." Together, over 200 community leaders and local residents developed recommendations for their neighborhoods that are both practical and actionable.[37] For instance,
  - o In a region of significant unemployment and underemployment, low-income households in New Orleans struggle to pay electric bills that are among the nation's highest. The report offers recommendations from community-based organizations and employers for bringing bills down and growing jobs.
  - o The average cost of owning a car in New Orleans is nearly $9,000 annually—which means taking public transportation can save families a lot of money and help reduce greenhouse gas emissions. However, the average transit-reliant New Orleanian can reach only 12 percent of jobs in the area within 30 minutes. The report recommends public transit improvements, such as expanded bus routes and more reliable schedules for underserved communities.

These recommendations are not pie-in-the-sky. Each requires partnerships and collaborations with key stakeholders across the city. In short, achieving equity and taking responsible action on climate change require all of us to work together.—Beverly Wright

Many of the collaborative principles and goals of the center are reflected in research presented at a 2019 *Sharing Knowledge* poster session by Romona Taylor Williams, executive director of North Montgomery Communities United for Prosperity in Mississippi. Called Achieving Sustainability Through Education

and Economic Development or ASEED, this two-year pilot project was established in Duck Hill, a small, majority low-wealth African-American community that has been plagued for decades by severe flooding and poor stormwater
infrastructure.

ASEED is designed to create a resident-driven community model that will
"lessen residents' vulnerability to climate-related disasters" while also developing citizen leaders to advance resilience and equity.[38] Funded through RWJF's
Integrative Action for Resilience program, ASEED specifically supports inter-
generational leadership development programs that help develop strong community leaders who can work toward positive economic, environmental, and
social justice outcomes.[39] According to Williams, ASEED has recruited 75 adult
leaders and trained 12 students, ages 12 to 18, to identify solutions to their
most pressing stresses. So far, the community has come together to install a
stormwater diversion system to mitigate severe flooding; worked to restore five
creeks in the Duck Hill community that contribute to flooding; and conducted a
climate vulnerability assessment. The teenage "Creek Rangers" have performed
creek cleanups, tested soil and water conditions, and installed rain gardens.

The work to mitigate climate change on a community level is daunting, Wright
admits, and sometimes the failures along the way are heartbreaking. "The state
of Louisiana," she says, "where Hurricane Katrina occurred in 2005, has now
experienced its first climate refugees, with members of the Biloxi-Chitimacha-
Choctaw community on the Isle de Jean Charles being relocated because of sea-
level rise."[40]

Despite such setbacks, all three experts say that progress has been made.

*Today, more and more people are aware of what we have been saying for the
last 40 years, which is this: if we don't make climate resilience that's equitable,
if we don't protect the least in our society, it's like a weak chain. If you don't
make the whole chain strong, the weakest link will bring the whole system
down.*—Robert Bullard

A Final Word

Through research, evaluation, and grantmaking, RWJF is engaged in multiple
efforts to address climate change and environmental justice as part of its commitment to a Culture of Health and health equity. These RWJF efforts include
looking at solutions from around the globe in search of lessons for improving
health, equity, and climate in U.S. cities[41] and supporting local initiatives in small
towns and Indigenous communities.

For example, through its Health and Climate Solutions program, RWJF has funded seven community initiatives that draw on local and Indigenous knowledge to address climate change[42]:

- **Buffalo, New York:** People United for Sustainable Housing, Inc. (PUSH) Buffalo is helping weatherproof houses to improve energy efficiency, community development, and resilience.
- **Portland, Oregon:** Friends of Trees is planting trees in low-income, ethnically diverse neighborhoods to enhance local health and well-being.
- **Anchorage, Alaska:** The Alaska Native Tribal Health Consortium has developed an innovative, portable water sanitation system for homes in rural, Native Alaskan communities where climate change impacts on infrastructure and the environment have made it nearly impossible to access safe, clean water.
- **Austin, Texas:** City officials, increasingly concerned about residents enduring extreme heat, are planting more trees to increase green space and shade around some of the city's public schools, especially those that largely serve students of color or lower income neighborhoods.
- **Finland, Minnesota, and Navajo communities, New Mexico:** The Swinomish Indian Tribal Community in Minnesota and Navajo communities in New Mexico are blending CDC recommendations for building resilience against climate effects with traditional Indigenous values, understanding, and practices. In both states, farmers are using crop rotation and innovative grazing practices—known as regenerative farming—to improve the quality of crops, foster soil health, and reduce the climate footprint of agriculture while improving the ability of crops to withstand flooding, drought, and heat.

Across the United States, people are recognizing that climate change is a major threat to any vision of a healthy future. They are responding by developing solutions.—RWJF, Health and Climate Solutions program

Spotlight

Multisolving to Advance Climate Goals

Elizabeth Sawin, PhD, Co-Founder and Co-Director, Climate Interactive

Experts invariably zero in on the health-damaging impacts of climate change in order to define the problem and drive change. But Elizabeth Sawin frames it differently.

A biologist with a PhD from the Massachusetts Institute of Technology, Sawin focuses on how attacking climate change can pay off with health dividends, and her strategy is to pursue climate and health goals at the same time. She and her colleagues at a nonprofit think tank called Climate Interactive describe this somewhat reverse approach with a word that Sawin invented—"multisolving," the potential for a single action or investment to solve multiple problems at once.

Multisolving at the Intersection of Health and Climate

When it comes to health and climate, multisolving means "helping people find solutions that reduce greenhouse gas emissions while producing multiple benefits in health, justice, resilience, equity, and well-being," according to the Climate Interactive website.[1]

Multisolving projects tend to commit to three principles, according to Sawin, writing in "The Magic of Multisolving," published in the Stanford Social Innovation Review[2]: Everyone matters, everyone is needed; addressing tough problems in an integrated fashion leads to success; and though large solutions start small, growth results from learning and connecting.

"One final ingredient for multisolving may be the most important of all: courage," she continues in her article. "It takes courage, especially in cultures that tend to value the strong, expert leader and the quick fix, to use this approach."

Elizabeth Sawin, *Spotlight: Multisolving to Advance Climate Goals* In: *Community Resilience*. Edited by: Alonzo L. Plough, Oxford University Press (2021). © Robert Wood Johnson Foundation. DOI: 10.1093/oso/9780197559383.003.0018

Consider these health and climate multisolving examples from a Climate Interactive 2018 report,[3] funded in part by the Robert Wood Johnson Foundation (RWJF):

Replacing a coal-fired power plant located in a highly populated area with a source of clean, renewable energy would reduce CO_2 emissions (climate benefit) while also improving air quality and reducing respiratory illnesses (health benefit).

Building a community garden in a low-income neighborhood would increase access to healthy foods (health benefit) while reducing CO_2 emissions from transporting food (climate benefit).

Investing in green space for urban stormwater management helps protect against the expected impact of more intense rainfall (climate benefit) while providing opportunities for recreation, exercise, and community connection (health benefit).

"Approaching climate change as a single issue has failed," asserts Sawin. "The reason multisolving is important is because we've been defining climate change too narrowly."

We have to remake our world in order to meet climate goals, and the opportunity to do that in a way that improves health, equity, and the livability of neighborhoods, while addressing social determinants of health, is huge.—Elizabeth Sawin

En-ROADS

A climate solutions simulation tool called En-ROADS, developed by Climate Interactive, allows people to discover what policies and investments will be needed to address climate change. En-ROADS scenarios help decision-makers understand all the ways that energy systems, the built environment, forestry, and food production will need to change to avoid the most dangerous impacts of climate change. These scenarios provide a jumping-off point for conversations about the health advantages and other benefits of those changes.

One of the biggest surprises in Sawin's work dates back to 2009, when she and a colleague discovered the literature showing that the health benefits derived from meeting climate change goals equaled, or exceeded, any of the costs associated with implementing change (a finding reinforced nearly 10 years later by the World Health Organization).[4]

"I had spent the previous 15 years of my life trying to convince people that addressing climate change for the future was going to cost money, going to be a sacrifice, but we had to do it. And then I discover, 'By the way, we're going to save

about as much money as it's going to cost.' From that moment, I felt like the world needed to better understand the size and scale of these co-benefits, of multisolving."

Climate Interactive is studying 10 international cases of multisolving for climate and health—cases that also provide economic, safety, and community improvement benefits. Among them are a program that switches hospitals to using anesthetic gases to lower costs and emissions; a healthy streets program in an international city that improves air quality, reduces congestion, and makes the city healthier and more attractive; and a campaign that encourages parents, teachers, and students to walk to school.

The good news is that multisolving solutions are emerging. People are finding ways to join hearts and minds into a different way of working together, making new solutions possible.—Elizabeth Sawin

ANALYTICAL FRAMEWORKS THAT DRIVE INNOVATION

Beginning with reflections on the role of narrative in shaping our world-view, this volume has confronted the many challenges to resilience and well-being as well as the inequity that so pervades the systems we rely on and the environments in which we live. Through stories of determination and commitment, presented in tandem with confirming data, it has also uncovered strategies for tackling obstacles in a spirit of realistic optimism.

In support of these ongoing efforts, this closing part directs attention to new methods of data collection and analyses. As they go beyond traditional models, these approaches demand a fresh kind of rigor, a thorough consideration of consequences, and a commitment to iterative learning.

As explored in chapter 13, "Digital Data, Ethical Challenges," ever-evolving technological advances offer the ability to investigate previously impenetrable topics, collect vast amounts of data from large numbers of people, include previously excluded groups in research, and gain new insights to inform policy and action. As this technology progresses, academic and industry researchers, designers, and strategists are diving deeper into a new digital world, with all of its potential and pitfalls. While the promised benefits are considerable, important concerns about informed consent, unintended consequences, and bias must be sensitively deliberated so that data use is fair, appropriate, and broadly beneficial.

In chapter 14, "Investing in Social Determinants: Fresh Perspectives on the Returns," contributors consider ways to measure financial and other returns from investing in interventions designed to bolster social determinants of health at the community level. An industrial and operations engineer, an economist, and an attorney examine the savings that accrue from removing leaded drinking water service lines and lead paint hazards, early childhood education programs, and other ventures. They also consider the role of Medicaid as a coordinator of financing for sustainable investments that help support the concept of "whole-person care." Managed by community-based organizations, these innovative efforts are yielding significant financial savings along with improved health and social outcomes.

Data provide the foundation for the evidence that can most productively direct energy, attention, and resources toward health and well-being. Careful analysis of the financial impact of such efforts will further enable the efficient use of resources and promote interventions most likely to generate positive outcomes. This final part of the book lifts up the innovation taking place in data collection and financial analysis, closing the volume with the conviction that we can make the right choices to secure a healthier future for all.

Digital Data, Ethical Challenges

Sara Holoubek, MBA, CEO, Luminary Labs

*Camille Nebeker, EdD, MS, Associate Professor, Family Medicine
and Public Health, School of Medicine, University of California,
San Diego; Co-Founder and Director, Research Center for
Optimal Digital Ethics—Health (ReCODE.Health)*

*Paul Tarini, MA, Senior Program Officer, Robert Wood Johnson
Foundation*

The imperative of resilience, and its fundamental role in building a Culture of
Health, is a core theme in this volume. As ideas for future policy and practice
to shape a more resilient and healthier society are developed, they must be
accompanied by new approaches to gathering the evidence that documents their
value. Innovation and inclusiveness are key here: Well-crafted biomedical and
behavioral research must go beyond traditional strategies, engage a richer set of
voices, and bring in novel sources of data. Rapidly expanding technology makes
much of this possible, giving us new ability to investigate previously impenetrable topics, bring new voices to the fore, and inform the narratives that shape
our lives.

Unlike traditional laboratory studies, pervasive sensor technologies (e.g.,
smartphones, Fitbits, iPads, and other devices that collect and transmit a range
of information easily and quickly) make it easier to obtain data from people as
they engage in routine activities. As a result, fresh opportunities for study and
analysis are emerging, bringing powerful insights about individual and community characteristics, strengths, and vulnerabilities that can inform policy and action. At the same time, introducing those health technologies in research raises
many questions: How will data be collected? Who owns them and with whom
will they be shared?

Sara Holoubek, Camille Nebeker, and Paul Tarini, *Digital Data, Ethical Challenges* In: *Community Resilience.*
Edited by: Alonzo L. Plough, Oxford University Press (2021). © Robert Wood Johnson Foundation.
DOI: 10.1093/oso/9780197559383.003.0019

How Will Data Interface With Existing Clinical Records?

The three contributors to this chapter help sort out the features of this remarkable new digital world. Sara Holoubek brings her experience as CEO and founder of Luminary Labs, a strategy and innovation consultancy that works with corporate, nonprofit, and government organizations. Camille Nebeker approaches these issues from an academic perspective, having developed the Research Center for Optimal Digital Ethics (ReCODE) at the University of California, San Diego. Robert Wood Johnson Foundation's (RWJF's) Paul Tarini offers insight from the foundation's decade-plus commitment to identifying and promoting technology that can advance people's ability to lead healthy lives. All agree that while there is much to embrace with enthusiasm, there is also good reason to proceed with cautious attention. Nebeker's "Spotlight: The HUMAN Project—Using Megadata to Analyze Health" at the end of this chapter offers an eye-opening look at the vast scope of data that are potentially available for analysis.

Confronting a New World

A University of California, San Diego (UCSD) researcher designed a study asking healthy volunteers to wear an outward-facing camera for a week, along with an accelerometer that measures physical activity and a GPS device to track location. The goal, as described by UCSD colleague Camille Nebeker, was to collect data on when and where participants were active or sedentary. But when the researcher brought her design before the university's institutional review board (IRB), it was turned down because a wearable camera would photograph people *near* the participant who had not consented to having their image included as part of the research record. (The National Research Act of 1974 and the establishment of the Federal Policy for the Protection of Human Research Subjects led to the requirement that research on human subjects must be approved by an IRB.[1,2] These are committees within institutions that review proposals for federally funded research to ensure that the rights, welfare, and well-being of human participants are safeguarded. The concept of informed consent is a key IRB concern.)

Where the researcher saw an opportunity to use a tool that did not depend on often-unreliable self-reports, the IRB saw a threat to consent and privacy. The new world of digital data is turning long-standing assumptions and practices upside down—and it is not at all clear that the world of health care and research is ready for it. By harnessing the power of technology, the field strives to deliver more efficient, personalized, and targeted health care. But perplexing challenges accompany this power, and the field is still trying to sort out myriad emerging ethical issues.

A range of devices, the data collected by those devices, and the ways in which the data are used are all components of this novel environment, according to RWJF's Paul Tarini. For example:

- A mobile phone app boosts medication adherence by providing reminders.
- Algorithms assess a person's computer keystrokes and smartphone swipes to detect potential markers for Parkinson's disease.
- Twitter data are used to identify disease outbreaks even before the Centers for Disease Control and Prevention (CDC) becomes aware of them.
- An asthma inhaler used by Air Louisville in Kentucky is equipped with a sensor that tracks when, where, and how often it is used, helping patients manage their symptoms and better control their asthma.

The personal devices that make all of this, and much more, possible are many and varied, including smartphones, credit cards, and wearables (e.g., smartwatches, fitness trackers, and tech-enabled clothing). The "internet of things" allows appliances, security systems, and lighting and speaker systems to collect, send, and act on the data they gather from the environment. The use of texting technology, which creates an avenue through which confidential assistance can be provided to people in emotional crises (see "Spotlight: Texting Through a Crisis," at the end of Chapter 7) is another example.

The tools used to capture personal health data nowadays are pervasive and ubiquitous.—Camille Nebeker

The data exist in standard computer language and are easy to copy without loss of fidelity. They can be deeply granular, yet readily stored and analyzed. "Ultimately, you can have much more data for analysis that can produce more insight," Tarini stresses. At the same time, these new types of data can be very complex, requiring similarly complex analyses.

This ever-evolving technology promises to expand both the scale and reach of research. Many more people can be included in a data set than could realistically have been included in a traditional study. Data can be collected in real world, nonlaboratory settings and on things for which information was previously unavailable.

The promise with digital data is the ability to have a deeper, richer, wider, more democratized dataset and be able to analyze it and develop more insights.—Paul Tarini

Studying Humans "in the Wild"

A further advantage of digital data collection tools is that they allow people to be observed in real time in their natural environment, without relying on their recall of events and self-reports, observes Nebeker. Since data are collected passively and unobtrusively, a continuous data stream is possible. In addition, as the tools become less expensive, the cost of data collection decreases.

People enrolled in large "virtual studies," as they are sometimes called, generally can control which data, such as heart rate or fitness activities, will be transmitted to researchers. Data are gathered as people engage in their regular activities, so participant burden is significantly reduced.

With digital research in the smart and connected environment we can monitor people 24/7, on the fly, in real time.—Camille Nebeker

Advancing Equity

The ability to capture data remotely also enables people who may not otherwise be adequately represented to be included in research; these could include those for whom travel to a clinic or research center would be difficult or impossible, such as people lacking appropriate and affordable transportation, living in rural regions, or who have disabilities. Their experiences and voices can help samples be more representative of the overall population and allow factors affecting the health of specific populations, such as race and ethnicity, to be more fully explored.

Beyond the research benefits, the techniques of digital health are "incredibly helpful for communities where access to health care is challenging," Nebeker emphasizes. Clinical expertise can be brought electronically to patients in isolated areas who are underserved by health professionals or to people for whom the logistics of accessing health care are time consuming and complicated. In addition, technology "can bring down the cost of care significantly," notes Tarini.

But against this backdrop, with all of its promise, lies a host of unanswered questions and looming concerns about how data will be collected, analyzed, and operationalized in health care delivery.

New Worries, New Challenges

We are not ready for the world we have programmed. Maybe we should slow down and think.—Sara Holoubek

The sea change that is the digital age is sweeping health and health care into its wake. In November 2019 the Harvard School of Public Health announced the new Apple Women's Health Study, designed to enroll one million women over 10 years. One of three large research projects being carried out by major academic centers and health organizations in conjunction with Apple, the study uses Apple iPhones and apps to enroll participants and collect data. It's a powerful partnership. Indeed, the *New York Times* called Apple's involvement in health research "the latest example of how the biggest tech companies are edging their way into the country's $3.5 trillion health care market."[3]

The advent of the private sector into health research is changing the landscape. As companies with access to large amounts of consumer data, such as Google, Apple, and Facebook, develop increasingly sophisticated analytic tools, important questions arise about how they will collect and use personal information. To begin, do the ethical and legal principles that typically guide the collection of health data in other research settings even apply?

This is uncharted territory, at least in part because even the definition of health data has become murky. "If it was collected from an app that may or may not have anything to do with health—yet something might be inferred about health—is it then health data?" asks Holoubek, adding that there are "no prevailing rules or guidelines" for collecting real-world evidence. And "if there is no framework for handling the data then there generally is no ethical framework."

Many large consumer-facing tech companies are concluding that any data used for a health purpose can indeed be considered health data and that if they don't take the lead on how it is used, government regulators may step in and decide for them. Moreover, companies that partner with academic researchers must meet IRB standards in order for those researchers to use the company-collected data. Private companies need to get "smart very quickly about how those data should be protected," says Holoubek. "They are realizing that they need to create that infrastructure."

In a departure from academic norms, companies may take health-related products shown to work in scientific literature, put them onto a software platform, and sell them as apps, without testing whether they are as effective in that format. While new testing would be expected in an academic setting to claim effectiveness, the private sector may ignore that additional task and just promote the product as effective. Nebeker acknowledges that some companies strive to do the right thing, especially when their leaders have an academic training in ethics and responsible practices. But others may be business-focused people who lack that ethical acculturation and decision-making framework as they pursue opportunities to bring innovative products to market.

While agreeing that the private sector at times may focus only on the promise of a new product or service, giving little attention to the "what-ifs" that underscore ethical concerns, Holoubek argues that a better future is possible.

I believe you can be both pro-tech and pro-ethics at the same time.—Sara Holoubek

An Ethical Framework

The National Commission for the Protection of Human Subjects of Biomedical and Behavioral Research, which drove the creation of IRBs, as described previously, issued its final report in 1978. Widely known as the Belmont Report, it identified three fundamental ethical principles that should underlie research on human subjects and established research guidelines consistent with those principles.[4]

Nebeker believes that the core principles defined in the Belmont Report remain applicable as an ethical framework for the digital age:

- **Respect for persons**—providing the information a person needs to make an informed decision to participate in research as a willing volunteer. In research involving data from digital devices, potential participants may not understand the details of the data collection. "Researchers and IRBs also may not sufficiently understand the technology used to gather data nor how to manage the data, which makes conveying information to the potential participant even more difficult," says Nebeker.
- **Beneficence**—weighing the benefits and risks of research participation, maximizing potential benefits, and minimizing potential harms. An individual's data and research literacy can affect risk assessment. Nebeker cautions that "in digital health, there are unknown unknowns that need to be considered with the help of experts."
- **Justice**—focusing on whether the participants are, or are representative of, those who are likely to benefit the most. This principle ensures that the knowledge gained from a study will help people like those in the study. Concern about bias in artificial intelligence (discussed in material that follows) stems from this principle.

The 2012 Menlo report, produced by cybersecurity experts with the U.S. Department of Homeland Security, proposed an ethical framework for information and communication technologies, or ICT, research grounded in the three principles described in the Belmont Report and added a fourth principle,[5] as follows:

- **Respect for law and public interest**—ensuring transparency of methodologies and results, along with accountability for actions. An example, Nebeker suggests, is the ability to access artificial intelligence training data "to look for bias and for the potential implications on humanity that need to be considered."

They're My Data—or Are They?

Any research on human subjects carries ethical responsibilities, but experts across sectors, from academia to industry, fear that the ethical issues surfacing in a digital world are not being adequately considered. Holoubek put these concerns into "a few buckets," which tie back to the Belmont Report principles:

- "Did I agree for these data to be collected about me?"
- "Did I consent to somebody else using my data?"
- "Am I aware of the unintended consequences? Are you [who collected my data] aware of the unintended consequences?"
- "How long are the data kept?"

Holoubek distilled these into one overarching question: "When I give my data, or if my data are taken without my consent, are the individuals or companies collecting those data thinking in my best interest?"

The uneven distribution of digital knowledge and savvy adds to the concern about the impact on marginalized populations. People who have historically been discriminated against and those who are older or lack internet access may be particularly susceptible to having their data used improperly, Holoubek cautions.

Law and regulation covering privacy, security, and risk in some arenas do not always apply to digital data. For example, the Health Insurance Portability and Accountability Act (HIPAA), the federal law governing how personal health information is handled, does not cover consumer devices like Fitbit even though the data they generate are "potentially relevant for understanding health status," observes Tarini. "You bump into this bifurcated world between HIPAA and research studies on the one hand and consumer space on the other."

Holoubek points out that the U.S. Food and Drug Administration (FDA) has established standards for tolerable risk (i.e., the level of risk acceptable to society) as they apply to the development and approval of a new drug, but is only (as of November 2020) in the early stages of piloting a digital health software precertification program as part of its Digital Health Innovation Action Plan.[6]

"We haven't yet agreed upon the tolerable level of risk when you're trying out something in the digital space," she observes.

Informed Consent

The ability to give informed consent to participate in research requires that individuals have the information they need to make knowledgeable decisions and the data, technology, and research literacy "to understand what they're getting into," Nebeker stresses. While some populations are especially limited in their level of literacy, anyone can have difficulty fully comprehending the details of a study and the use of the data. Nebeker believes that education would help, but that adds cost.

Holoubek zeroed in on an inherent lack in the system: "We have been conditioned to just check the box, and consumer internet companies have not been held accountable for the level of informed consent required of health data collection or usage. You have to tell people what could possibly go wrong."

Like Nebeker, Holoubek is a proponent of education to aid informed consent, with materials written at a fourth-grade reading level. "Companies need to be very clear about intended use; but rarely is the use specific in a digital application," she says. They also need to be transparent about who they are sharing data with, what rights participants have, what will happen with the data, and who owns the data and for how long.

Unintended Consequences

With these technologies comes the responsibility of imagining the unintended consequences.—Sara Holoubek

Technology is moving so quickly from generating an idea to deploying a solution that potential pitfalls are sometimes not fully considered. Holoubek stresses the need at all levels of an organization—from designer, developer, and business strategist to CEO and board member—to imagine unintended consequences. "When considering how your business is going to change courtesy of anything digital that can collect data, you also have to consider what could possibly go wrong. Unfortunately, this is playing out case by case, unintended consequence by unintended consequence."

An oft-cited example is that of the fitness app Strava, which published a global heat map of people running, walking, and cycling all over the world, based on user data. In doing so, they unwittingly uncovered secret military bases, including some in Iraq and Syria, at which service members were using Strava to record their runs. Strava "is sitting on a ton of data that most intelligence entities would literally kill to acquire," warned Jeffrey Lewis, PhD, of the Middlebury Institute of International Studies at Monterey.[7] Holoubek wonders: "Did anyone think about what could possibly happen if the data were made public?" Strava subsequently redesigned its app to address the issue, with the option to opt out of the global activities heat map feature now on the first page of user privacy settings. Users may also set up "privacy zones" that are not included in the maps.

Bias in Collecting and Using Digital Data

Bias—whether based on gender, race, ethnicity, socioeconomic status, or some other characteristic—can be introduced in the collection and use of digital data through both hardware and software.

Skewed Samples

Inadequate sampling can distort results. For example, studies designed to collect data from a Fitbit or an iPhone do not represent the general population because they only include users of those devices in their samples. The median income of iPhone users in the United States is about $89,000, while that of Android users is $64,510,[8] so a study that includes only iPhone users will skew to higher income, which needs to be factored into the study's statistical design. Other disparities may not even be known and so could introduce undetected bias into the results.

Algorithmic Bias

As treatment and health coverage decisions increasingly depend on computer algorithms, the bias of those algorithms is a significant issue. Artificial intelligence requires enough data so that a machine can be trained to understand patterns and start learning. If the training data set is not representative of the population being addressed, or is biased in some other way, that bias will be reflected in the results. "Algorithms fed with big data can replicate existing biases at a speed and scale that can create irreparable harm," wrote Holoubek and colleague Jessica Hibbard.[9] "If what we're feeding in is biased, what's coming out will be biased," Holoubek emphasizes. "And the minute you are making health-related recommendations, a life can literally be at risk."

As the system moves more and more to a backbone that is digitized and machine-learning- and artificial-intelligence-enabled, there is the risk that some of the current inequities in the system will get baked in. That's a real concern to us at RWJF.—Paul Tarini

In developing the training data set for a particular application, the developer must "consider every aspect to ensure that it is representative of the population," Holoubek emphasizes. Sample size alone is not enough. While a study of one million people providing real-time data from their iPhones is certainly large, it is not necessarily representative or unbiased. Holoubek describes "fierce debates among experts between what a randomized controlled trial to avoid bias should look like for digital medicine and whether researchers can just rely on real-world evidence."

Taking a broad view, Tarini emphasizes that the bias problem is not just limited to insufficiently representative data being built into algorithms. "It has to do with how we decide to use the data and for what purposes; the questions we're asking; the assumptions made about people, their health, the care they need, and how they use the health care system; and many other issues." As an example, a word pattern recognition algorithm underlying an Amazon engineer recruitment tool—built on a comparison of résumés of successful Amazon engineers (predominantly White males) over a 10-year period—led to the filtering out of women's résumés.[10] In an example of racial bias, the COMPAS (Correctional Officer Management Profiling for Alternative Sanctions) algorithm used by judges in detain or release-on-bail decisions discriminated against Black defendants. Black defendants were incorrectly labeled as likely to commit future crimes at almost twice the rate as Whites. Likewise, Whites were incorrectly labeled as being at low risk for committing future crimes more frequently than Blacks.[11]

Nebeker is a member of the Committee for Scientific Freedom and Responsibility of the American Association for the Advancement of Science, which launched a three-year exploration of artificial intelligence and ethics in 2018. The head of the National Institute of Standards and Technology, a standards development group, reported to the committee that the institute has made a commitment not to use training data without factoring in the risk for bias and considering the potential damage to particular populations. Nebeker lauds their commitment but cautions that "not all are setting high standards." While several bills focused on the regulation of artificial intelligence are pending before Congress and there is increasing attention to the topic at other levels of government, she concedes that it would take some time to address the issue fully.

For a case study of the benefits, risks, and ethical issues involved in collecting and using digital data, see "Spotlight: The HUMAN Project—Using Megadata to Analyze Health" at the end of this chapter.

What's to Be Done?

In ethics, there are few easy answers. The digital age brings new ethical challenges and unknown unknowns.—Camille Nebeker

Five strategies are key to advancing the ethical collection and use of digital data to realize promising health benefits without compromising individual privacy and security: commitment, education, inclusion, infrastructure, and regulation.

Commitment

Holoubek describes "two thoughts on digital ethics: the armchair philosophers who are the historical guardians of ethics and the lawyers." She believes the right strategies draw on "an understanding from both of these parties, but, more importantly, for the people in the business to actually care."

Some companies have ethical oaths that leaders and employees are expected to respect, but many do not. Holoubek recommends that companies create a code of ethics for data science and technology and make a commitment to institutionalize ethics within their organizations. For support, she offered the Ethical OS Toolkit, a framework created jointly by the Institute for the Future and the Omidyar Network that identifies "risk zones" and strategies for taking ethical action.[12] As well, the Digital Health Framework and Checklist from ReCODE Health, described in material that follows, supports decision-making by researchers with a goal of protecting research participants, Nebeker notes.[13]

Education

Whoever is involved—developer, designer, business strategist—and whatever they are considering (a potential solution, a study, a therapy) that results in additional data, the question that must be asked is, "What is the worst possible thing that could happen?" The answer should mediate the continued development of any new tool.

Ethics-based training, such as ways to detect algorithmic bias, would broaden the perspective of those tasked with technological development. Holoubek's suggestion for helping to think about the ethical ramifications of new technology is to assign greater value to broad-based education and the liberal arts and to tone down the "bro" culture of some programming:

> *Less brogrammer, more Leonardo da Vinci. Read more fiction and watch more movies. These will hone one's ability to anticipate unintended consequences.*—Sara Holoubek

Inclusion

Companies should foster work teams that are diverse by gender, race, ethnicity, age, and other characteristics, and that draw on many academic disciplines and backgrounds so that different lived experiences, ideas, and types of thinking can be brought to bear on the "worst possible thing" question. "All members must have the ability to speak up and be listened to in the same way," stresses Holoubek. Support for dissent throughout the organization is critical and adds to ethical protections.

Infrastructure

Investment in infrastructure will help ensure that institutions and companies have the support framework they need to consider and implement systems for ethical data collection and use. But funders all too often prefer to support " 'sexy science' and not boring infrastructure," says Nebeker.

At the University of California, San Diego, Nebeker and colleagues have used RWJF funding to establish the Connected and Open Research Ethics (CORE) platform, which is a key feature of ReCODE. ReCODE supports technologists, researchers, ethicists, regulators, institutions, and participants in digital health research to increase awareness of ethical principles and practices at every step of the research process, beginning with the initial design.[14] In addition to providing the community with decision support tools, the CORE platform hosts a resource library and a forum that connects researchers and allows users to pose questions to experts.[15]

Regulation

The limited regulations that currently exist are inconsistent, according to Nebeker. To put appropriate regulation in place, Holoubek believes, more elected officials are needed who are digital natives (i.e., grew up in the digital age) or are both technologically and ethically fluent. "That's probably 20 years out," admits Holoubek, who also predicts that regulation is coming.

RWJF's Dive Into Digital Health

More than a decade ago, RWJF's Pioneer Team—the group tasked with uncovering developing trends that have potentially big impacts on people's health—took notice of the emerging class of real-world, real-time data and began to fund initiatives that could use these data to advantage. As Tarini relates, this started with *Project HealthDesign*[16] in 2006, which explored how activities of daily living can contribute to personal health records and provide clinicians with a more comprehensive picture of their patients' lives.

Later, a 2013 RWJF grant to Sage Bionetworks looked at creating an open platform for science focused on what patients need and how they think. That effort, Tarini notes, "pivoted into work that helped produce Apple's ResearchKit," which is an online framework for collecting data for medical research.[17] These and many other projects, including the work of Camille Nebeker and her colleagues at ReCODE,[18] helped the foundation establish a rich base of knowledge and experience.

More recently, RWJF funded the *Fairness in Precision Medicine* project in 2018 led by Data & Society, which looked at how the field of precision medicine is unfolding, identified potential problems with fairness and bias, and made recommendations for avoiding those problems.[19] In 2019, the foundation made seven grants under a new program, *Exploring the Influence of Technology on Health*, which looks at "ways that the data-rich world we are moving into will enable change that has all kinds of health consequences, on the individual level and on the community level," says Tarini.

RWJF's immersion in the new technology continues. Tarini summarizes the journey as going from grappling with brand new concepts to having concrete cases that can help determine how to mitigate the potential harms of technology and optimize its public and personal benefits.

A Final Word

The explosion in digital data raises ethical issues that confront both academic and industry researchers as they explore health behaviors, environmental factors, and the social circumstances of individuals and populations. Use of these data provides opportunities to develop a deeper understanding of the influences on people's health and their ability to access the full range of supports needed to live the healthiest lives possible.

But it imposes responsibilities as well. From making sure that research participants are fully informed, to rooting out algorithmic bias that can substantially impact the care people receive, to keeping data private and ensuring an ethical approach to its collection and use, thoughtful commitment is needed from all involved. This may translate into concrete actions, such as funding research on the ethical, legal, and social implications of digital health research and practice; including a health technology ethicist on study teams; and bringing diverse consumer voices into the early design of health technology applications. To take full advantage of the potential this new world holds, nothing less will suffice.

Spotlight

The HUMAN Project—Using Megadata to Analyze Health

Camille Nebeker, EdD, MS, Associate Professor, Family Medicine and Public Health, School of Medicine, University of California, San Diego; Co-Founder and Director, Research Center for Optimal Digital Ethics—Health (ReCODE.Ḥealth)

The HUMAN Project was initiated in 2014 by the Kavli Foundation in partnership with New York University's Institute for the Interdisciplinary Study of Decision Making.[1] Its goal was to collect vast amounts of data from a representative sample of 10,000 New York City residents in 4,000 households over 20 years. Lacking both internal review board approval and sustainable funding, the ḤUMAN Project was suspended in 2018. Nonetheless, the ambitious scope of the study and what it revealed about the possibilities for collecting and using data in the digital age are intriguing. It is possible that this type of model could eventually be revived, perhaps with additional privacy protections built in.

The scope of the initiative is reflected in the virtually endless list of data sources on which these pioneers intended to draw: financial records, surveys, genomic testing, electronic health records, social network data, phone and text messages, search strategies, criminal justice data, GPS data, family networks, household movement detectors, wearable devices, and more. "These data sources, when brought together, can be used to infer personal health status," says Camille Nebeker, who served on the project's Ethics Advisory Council.

The possible study questions are equally vast. Researchers would have been able to request access to the secure data set for virtually any health or public policy question, from Alzheimer's disease, public transit, and education to mental health, nutrition, and affordable housing. The intent, says Nebeker, was to bring the disparate and siloed data together "to make sense of human health." Potential users would include not only academic scholars, but also insurance companies, tech companies, and many others.

Camille Nebeker, *Spotlight: The HUMAN Project—Using Megadata to Analyze Health* In: *Community Resilience*. Edited by: Alonzo L. Plough, Oxford University Press (2021). © Robert Wood Johnson Foundation. DOI: 10.1093/oso/9780197559383.003.0020

The HUMAN Project gets people to think about the possibilities of using existing data to better understand what's happening in human health.—Camille Nebeker

The Ethics Advisory Council was convened to ensure the privacy and security of the data and provide guidance on ethical, legal, and social implications of the project. Although data are supposed to be de-identified, participant anonymity was not actually guaranteed. Moreover, because these studies were to evolve over time, a participant would have no way of knowing what the data would ultimately be used for after they consented to participate, raising the issue of whether consent could truly be informed.

All of that only hints at the potential benefits and risks of collecting and analyzing wide-ranging and detailed personal data from individuals over time. The ability to predict disease patterns, the availability of data presumably more accurate than self-reported data, and the generalizability of data from a representative sample are examples of benefits the study would offer.

At the same time, barriers to comprehensive informed consent, the potential for discrimination resulting from genomic testing, the likely lack of anonymity, and the drawing in of others who are not participants—say, visitors picked up on household sensors—are all issues to be examined carefully and prospectively to identify and mitigate potential risks and enhance the benefits of any knowledge gained. These and other ethical concerns, such as who owns the data and who can benefit financially from its use, are ripe for discussion.

‖ 14 ‖

Investing in Social Determinants

Fresh Perspectives on the Returns

Lynn A. Karoly, PhD, Senior Economist, Professor, Pardee RAND Graduate School, RAND Corporation

Cindy Mann, JD, Partner, Manatt Health, Manatt, Phelps & Phillips

George Miller, PhD, Institute Fellow, Center for Value in Health Care, Altarum

The emerging consensus that steep investments in high-end clinical care have not yielded commensurate improvements in patient outcomes is a cornerstone of the Robert Wood Johnson Foundation's (RWJF's) commitment to building a Culture of Health. So, too, is the recognition that a lack of upstream investments in prevention and social services have left some of the most significant contributors to poor health unattended. As interest grows in understanding the complex interactions between social needs and well-being, pioneering work is demonstrating that the right interventions can prevent costly and debilitating health problems downstream, yielding a reasonable return on investment (ROI) in the form of future cost savings.

The contributors to this chapter—an industrial and operations engineer, an economist, and an attorney—draw on their work to illustrate the value of addressing the causes of poor health at their roots. Combining business principles of ROI with outcome data from social interventions, they argue that addressing social determinants not only builds resilience and improves health but also yields savings that may accrue to health, social, and other systems.

Suggesting that approaching social interventions as "nonclinical prevention" sharpens understanding of investments and outcomes, George Miller describes Altarum's Value of Health tool as a strategy for determining ROI.

Lynn A. Karoly, Cindy Mann, and George Miller, *Investing in Social Determinants* In: *Community Resilience.*
Edited by: Alonzo L. Plough, Oxford University Press (2021). © Robert Wood Johnson Foundation.
DOI: 10.1093/oso/9780197559383.003.0021

Early childhood interventions can improve outcomes *and* save money, according to the RAND Corporation's Lynn A. Karoly. Her extensive studies of a range of interventions, in collaboration with other RAND colleagues, point to key short- and long-term health, social, and economic impacts.

Cindy Mann, a partner at Manatt, Phelps & Phillips, which provides legal and other professional services, presents the case for Medicaid as a player in addressing social needs because it covers beneficiaries with complex challenges, absorbs a significant share of the costs when these challenges are poorly addressed, and plays a key role in setting health policy. She describes evolving developments in North Carolina as a case example.

Creating the Value Proposition

At Altarum, a nonprofit research and consulting organization designed to advance health among vulnerable and publicly insured populations, George Miller studies opportunities to make health care spending in the United States more sustainable.

Miller's early work used mathematical modeling to examine the role of clinical prevention in improving health and managing health care costs. But colleagues began to suggest that "we were looking at the wrong kind of prevention," he says, explaining his shift in focus. "We needed to be talking not about clinical prevention but about social determinants of health."

Making the case for that kind of investing means demonstrating that "nonclinical prevention" does more than yield better health outcomes and reduce inequity. It should also be financially viable, returning benefits of importance to individuals, governments, and businesses. But developing evidence of economic benefit can be difficult for several reasons:

- It is often hard to quantify the economic impact of social problems such as food insecurity or delayed childhood development.
- There is a long horizon, often years, between an investment and its payoff.
- The system that makes the investment may not be the one that realizes the return, known as the "wrong-pockets problem."

"Value of Health" Tool Informs Policy and Practice

Through a series of grants from RWJF, Miller and his team developed the Value of Health tool to measure the costs and benefits of clinical and social interventions.[1]

Those investments "have eventual impact in the form of changes in the health of the affected population, changes in health care costs and nonhealth effects, as well as changes in expenditures associated with the intervention itself," he says.

> *The intervention costs and the intervention impact on health care costs, disparities, and nonhealth factors give stakeholders a picture of what they get for what they buy.*—George Miller

The framework is designed to clarify the process by which an upstream investment realizes its returns.[2] The tool synthesizes data from literature and national data sets to describe the long-term impacts of prevention-oriented investments on earnings, health, incarceration, life expectancy, and other factors. By design, it presents the costs and benefits in terms that are of use to policymakers, businesses, and consumers.

Measuring the Savings From Reducing Childhood Exposure to Lead

The crisis that unfolded in the Flint, Michigan, water system, as well as ongoing reports of dangerous lead levels in other communities, offers a powerful example of how the Value of Health tool can be used. As part of a study of lead contamination for the Pew Charitable Trusts,[3] Miller and colleagues from Child Trends (a research organization focusing on improving the lives of young people) used the tool to assess the ROI from reducing children's exposure to lead.

The analysis is designed to measure lifelong impacts of interventions on a cohort of children born in the United States in 2018 and for additional children born into the same households over the next 10 years. Benefits were discounted at 3 percent per year to account for changes in the value of the dollar over time.

Key findings include the following:

- Removing 272,000 leaded drinking water service lines would cost about $2 billion and protect 350,000 children; cut blood lead levels by one-third; generate $2.7 billion in benefits, mostly from higher earnings and lower medical costs; and return up to $1.33 per dollar invested.
- Removing 244,000 lead paint hazards, such as peeling and chipping paint from older homes where children from low-income families live, would cost $2.5 billion and protect 311,000 low-income children; cut blood levels by 40 percent; generate $3.5 billion in benefits; and return up to $1.39 per dollar invested.
- Ensuring that contractors comply with Environmental Protection Agency (EPA) lead-safe renovation and repair standards would protect 211,000

children; generate $4.5 billion in benefits; and return up to $3.10 per dollar invested.

(See chapter 9: "Health Care Institutions Step Forward to Support Resilient Communities," for more on the value of preventing lead exposure risks.)

A Value of Lead Prevention Tool

The Value of Lead Prevention tool,[4] an interactive visualization of state-level results from the Value of Health tool, guides state officials in calculating the impact of lead exposure and remediation. For children born in 2019, the publicly available website (www.valueofleadprevention.org) estimates the number of at-risk children in each state, the percentage in each county, and the economic burdens of lead contamination. It also measures the benefits of interventions to reduce lead exposure on businesses and public sector budgets.

Work underway as of February 2020 will expand the Value of Lead Prevention tool, enabling stakeholders to calculate the ROI from reducing lead contamination in nine select cities. Here, Miller and Altarum staff have taken a hands-on approach, collaborating with city officials to ensure that the tool provides the most useful information possible.

Looking Ahead

As the momentum for investing in social determinants builds, so does the demand for investments that yield commensurate social and financial returns. The use of proxy or intermediate measures, such as improvements in school attendance or completion of job training, is one way to generate confidence that investments are on the right course, Miller believes.

Interest in social impact bonds, in which private investors fund a public sector intervention designed to achieve specified outcomes, has also grown in recent years. If the intervention works, the government repays the investor with interest; if not, the investor bears the loss. In permitting the use of social impact bonds for evidence-based maternal and early childhood programs, the Bipartisan Budget Act of 2018 spoke clearly to the increasing federal interest in this approach.

Another strategy under study, the Collaborative Approach to Public Good Investment (CAPGI), focuses on the role of partnerships in generating ROI. A project of the College of Health and Human Services at George Mason University, this is a financing model in which stakeholders jointly invest in an initiative from which they all stand to benefit, explains Miller, who is part of the CAPGI team. Tweaking a little-known economic model known as the Vickrey-Clarke-Groves model, which dates back to the 1970s,[5] CAPGI is a structured approach that draws on available data to demonstrate to each stakeholder in the collaborative that it is in their self-interest to pay for an intervention.

"This self-interest is what makes the intervention an investment, rather than a donation," wrote the authors of a 2018 *Health Affairs* article.[6] Investments are more likely than donations or grants to be sustainable over time, they argued. In June 2019, CAPGI invited coalitions, providers, government agencies, and others to participate in a feasibility study to test its approach and to provide technical assistance to some of them in 2020.

As new models continue to be tested, one facet of ROI that warrants future research, Miller maintains, is the interaction of various social determinants. For example, health is positively correlated with both income and education, and income and education are also positively correlated, making it hard to tease apart these complex associations.

The Case for Investing in Early Childhood

Quality early childhood experiences for vulnerable children offer another significant opportunity to achieve ROI, given the growing consensus that such investments are money well spent. "I don't have to spend as much time making the case," says RAND economist Lynn A. Karoly, reflecting on how awareness of the importance of promoting resilience among children has changed. "People really kind of get it." (See chapter 7: "Addressing Trauma and Building Resilience in Children: Science and Practice," for further insights about this population.)

Karoly has long been interested in policy-relevant work aimed at reducing inequity and in exploring how investments in human capital might alleviate poverty. With colleagues Jill S. Cannon, PhD, and M. Rebecca Kilburn, PhD, she shares a history of collaborative research in this area, and in 2017 released an RWJF-funded study, "Investing Early: Taking Stock of Outcomes and Economic Returns From Early Childhood Programs,"[7] the third in a series of studies over the past 20 years.

That study sought to answer three questions:

- What approaches to providing services to families and children from the prenatal period to school entry have been rigorously evaluated?
- What outcomes did these programs improve in the short and long term?
- What are the costs and benefits of effective programs and the returns to government and society?

What Approaches Have Been Rigorously Evaluated?

The meta-analysis synthesized a broad set of programs for intervening in children's lives, all of which met five criteria: They covered some period between the prenatal months and the end of prekindergarten (pre-K); served the child or the parent; measured at least one child outcome; operated in the United States; and featured a rigorous research design that allowed for causal inferences.

An extensive literature review yielded 115 programs that met these criteria. A big surprise, Karoly notes, "was that the number of programs that met our criteria for having rigorous evidence had increased so much since our last study in 2005."[8] Back then, only 20 programs met the criteria.

The 115 programs varied widely and in important ways. Most were small when evaluated, serving a median of 244 families. Some, such as universal pre-K, served all children within a geographical area, while others targeted certain groups, such as low-income or at-risk children and families. Collectively, they reported on 3,183 outcomes in behavior and emotion, cognitive achievement, child health, developmental delay, employment and earnings in adulthood, and other areas.

Programs were also diverse in their area of focus and type of service delivered, sorting out as follows:

- Traditional early care and education programs that serve children in group settings and aim to promote child development (35)
- Home visiting programs that provide services primarily to parents in their homes (30)
- Out-of-home individual or group parent education programs (18)
- Income transfer programs, such as child-care vouchers and public assistance (7)
- Programs that use a combination of two or more approaches (25)

Most programs were designed to provide services for less than one year (typical for early care and education and parent education programs), but 23 programs offered services for three years or more (typically programs with a home visiting component). Children and parents entered and exited the programs at different times, partly due to changes in personal circumstances (e.g., moving) and partly due to program design. For example, many home visiting programs begin before the child is born, while pre-K programs serve children starting at about age three.

All programs tracked children after they left the program, but here, too, there was significant variation. A hospital-based program serving children in neonatal intensive care followed them for a few months after discharge, while many center-based programs tracked children for as long as five to ten years after they left. A few collected follow-up data for much longer, sometimes decades and in at least one instance until participants reached age 40.

What Are Some Key Short- and Long-Term Outcomes?

The research team classified outcomes as favorable, null, or unfavorable. To be favorable or unfavorable, a program had to affect the measured child outcome at a statistical significance level of 5 percent or better (i.e., with 95% likelihood, the outcome would be different from zero). Using these classifications, they found the following:

- Of the 3,183 outcomes measured, 923 (29%) were favorable, "a much larger percent than one would expect from chance using a 5-percent significance level," reports Karoly. About 70 percent of outcomes were null, and about 1 percent were unfavorable.
- Three domains—behavior and emotion, cognitive achievement, and child health—accounted for 77 percent of all favorable outcomes.
- Most programs (102 of the 115) favorably affected at least one outcome. However, Karoly warns, "It is not necessarily the case that every program is a home run on all of the outcomes that get measured."

Analyses showed that outcomes endured over time, she adds. "It is noteworthy that the outcomes decades after the program ended are favorable at a rate similar to those closer to the time the program ended."

In a meta-analysis of three key health indicators, the RAND team found that effects on birth outcomes (weight, prematurity, and health at birth) were statistically significant but small, and that the effect on body mass index (BMI) measured in middle childhood was not significant. However, the effects on adolescent substance use were significant, even several years after the intervention. That compares favorably with outcomes from interventions that take place during adolescence itself.

What Are the Costs, Benefits, and Returns?

Although "economic evaluations still are not routinely conducted," says Karoly, there is a clear trend upward—25 programs in the latest synthesis included a formal economic evaluation, up from just seven in 2005. Of those, 19 had a benefit-cost analysis, measuring the total value of the outcomes compared with the estimate of program costs; four featured cost-effectiveness analyses, measuring the cost required for the program to produce a given outcome; and two collected cost data only.

"There is not an industry standard in terms of measures for particular outcomes," Karoly cautions, making it impossible to develop "apples-to-apples" comparisons across programs. Nonetheless, the team was able to analyze and draw observations from the financial data, adjusting their findings to 2016 dollars to examine the ROI.

Cost differences across the 25 programs reflected vast variations in program structure: frequency of the services (daily, weekly, or monthly); length of the program (months or years); and design (individual or group focused). A parent education program featuring three home visits, for example, cost $150 per family, compared with a full-time, year-round child development program provided over five years, which cost $48,800 per family.

Although the economic benefits varied widely as well, the ROI results are promising. Fully 75 percent of the 19 programs that included a benefit-cost analysis showed benefits to society exceeding costs. "Regardless of the low or high cost of the program, benefit-cost analyses show that positive economic returns are possible for a range of programs," Karoly concludes, noting favorable measures from shorter and longer programs, high- and low-intensity programs, and targeted and universal programs.

The typical rate of return was $2 to $4 return for every dollar invested, representing a double to quadruple return for each dollar of cost.—Lynn A. Karoly

Most of the benefits accrue to program participants themselves, often appearing as higher earnings in adulthood. Only two of the 13 programs that analyzed the returns to government found that the benefits to the public sector exceeded program costs.

Implications for Next Steps

The findings offer reason for optimism, giving policymakers and practitioners more confidence that early intervention builds resilience, improves children's lives, and yields financial gains to society that outweigh their costs. The increase in the number of programs with evaluations adds to the menu of evidence-based programs from which to choose.

Ascertaining the net long-term ROI from early childhood programs is still a new endeavor, however, and "there is considerable uncertainty in the estimates of longer-term economic returns," Karoly says. Until measures and methods are standardized, it will remain impossible to compare programs, but future research should be designed to do that so effective programs can be highlighted, funded, and replicated, Karoly and her colleagues recommend. A deeper look into "the black box" of effective programs, she says, "would tell us why they are working."

Government and private funders can add to the knowledge base by requiring that evaluations include ROI analyses and setting aside funds for that purpose. While this component is increasingly part of grant requirements, more can be done. Identifying further opportunities to publish ROI studies of social programs would also encourage wider discussion of methods and strategies that might apply across disciplines and subject matter.

The Next Generation of Medicaid

The interplay between social determinants of health and ROI is especially relevant to Medicaid both because it is a vast program—with nearly 64 million people enrolled as of January 2020[9]—and because it plays an outsized role in health care policy and reimbursement. Federal and state Medicaid spending totaled $597.4 billion in fiscal year 2018, accounting for 16 percent of national health expenditures that year.[10]

Concerns about rising costs and less-than-optimal outcomes across the health care system have led state Medicaid programs, health systems, and managed care officials to move into what Cindy Mann calls the "next generation of Medicaid," one that emphasizes high-value, whole-person care. Whole-person care, she says, means that "as a health provider, when I assess somebody I am evaluating and thinking about an action plan for comprehensively addressing the needs of that person."

As a former legal services attorney working in poor communities, then as a federal Medicaid official, and now as a partner at Manatt, Phelps & Phillips, Mann recognizes an opportunity to improve well-being and perhaps lower costs to Medicaid or other service systems by addressing homelessness, hunger, violence, and inequality. "Studies are important to evaluate what interventions are most effective and appropriate for investment by the health care system," she acknowledges. But, she added, "we don't need a lot of studies to tell us that what goes on in people's lives and in their neighborhoods affects their health."

Quality Services, Cost Effectiveness, and
Better Outcomes

A next-generation Medicaid program that provides whole-person care is one in which the following holds:

- Multidisciplinary care management teams, backed with training and decision support tools, embed social needs into their work and take a hands-on approach to help beneficiaries secure needed services.
- These teams employ evidence-based tools to systematically screen beneficiaries and identify those with unmet nonmedical needs. Screening requires authentic, trusted relationships and careful thought about the right screening tool and the best way to conduct the screening.
- A network of community-based organizations and the health care sector work together to bridge long-standing gaps between health and social services, moving beyond a system of making referrals to constructing an integrated network that spans service systems.
- Financing, including but not limited to Medicaid, is organized to support sustainable investment interventions addressing social needs typically provided by in community organizations. Medicaid may cover care coordination (including helping enrollees access other services), certain nonmedical benefits, some infrastructure development, and quality improvement initiatives. Health plans with Medicaid contracts have even greater flexibility to use their Medicaid dollars to provide nonmedical benefits (referred to as value-added services) of this type.

Comprehensive evaluations allow state agencies, managed care organizations, and health systems to demonstrate both clinical effectiveness and ROI, recognizing that for some enrollees, such as children, the returns may accrue to systems other than Medicaid, such as the child welfare or education systems, or they may accrue over a longer time horizon.

Earlier crises have thrust Medicaid into the forefront of health care innovation, social services, and cost containment. "Medicaid was the key payer for HIV/AIDS services, and really care moved forward for those with HIV/AIDS," Mann notes. "So, it is not surprising to me that in some respects Medicaid has also started to think more aggressively about how to integrate social needs into the delivery of health care."

Medicaid also "jumped into managed care starting in the 1990s," Mann says, and managed care is now a routine form of Medicaid delivery and reimbursement in most states. As of July 2019, 39 states plus the District of Columbia contract with managed care plans for all or some of their beneficiaries.[11] A system of managed care is not an essential ingredient for integrating social needs into health services, she notes, but it offers additional levers that state Medicaid programs can readily engage.

Another important impetus for adopting a whole-person approach is that Medicaid officials are increasingly holding health care providers and plans accountable for a range of outcomes, pressing them to identify community interventions that can improve care and reduce future costs within and outside the health care delivery system. "The financial impetus of a reformed payment system pushes stakeholders to look at those interventions," Mann says.

In some situations, Medicaid's financial interest is clear and compelling; for example, installing a home air conditioner can reduce asthma attacks. For a homeless adult, however, the needed interventions may be particularly costly and for some populations, such as children, the savings that accrue from community-based services are not as easily measured because the ROIs are not immediate and may accrue to other budgets. North Carolina is one state that has taken a comprehensive approach to examining benefits and costs across systems.

Improving Outcomes in North Carolina

North Carolina took a big step toward privileging health over health care when, in October 2018, the federal Centers for Medicare and Medicaid Services (CMS) approved the state's request to shift Medicaid to managed care with strong care management requirements and permitted the state to reimburse community agencies in pilot communities to be reimbursed for select nonmedical expenses. The state gained some attention for this shift in an August 2018 *Modern Healthcare* article, "Social Determinants of Health Are Core of North Carolina's Medicaid Overhaul."[12] While these initiatives have been delayed due to state budget issues, they are now back on track with the managed care component to begin in mid-2021.

North Carolina Medicaid wants to buy health, not health care.
—Cindy Mann

Resources for Health Care Plans and Providers

Some resources developed for Medicaid managed care plans have already been out in pace and will be available to any health plan and provider in North Carolina. These tools allow care management teams to identify unmet health-related needs, assist beneficiaries in meeting them, and capture data consistently.

One tool that will be available for broad statewide use, for example, is an electronic coordinated care network (NCCARE360), which is a resource directory backed up by health navigators and by text and chat options. A shared platform allows providers to seamlessly make referrals and obtain follow-up information, and an online request form allows beneficiaries to ask for assistance.

Special initiatives to be undertaken by Medicaid managed care plans under the waiver include greater integration of behavioral, physical, and pharmacy services; expanded access to treatment for addiction; and the Healthy Opportunities pilot sites. An external evaluation will track outcomes and the value of the care being delivered.

Healthy Opportunities Pilot Sites

Healthy Opportunities pilot projects in North Carolina, slated to start after the implementation of managed care, represent a significant departure from traditional Medicaid. Up to $650 million in Medicaid funding over five years is available to implement several regional pilots, each designed to improve health and social outcomes and help contain health care costs. Select services approved for the pilots address housing, food, transportation, and interpersonal safety.

Healthy Opportunities is not designed to be off on the side; it is designed to be embedded in the delivery of care.—Cindy Mann

In each pilot region, a community-based Healthy Opportunities lead pilot entity will serve a central coordinating role under a contract from the state. The entity will, in turn, contract with managed care plans and community-based organizations, serving as the interface between the two. It will also train and guide community organization staff in delivering services, hold them accountable for meeting program standards, collect and submit data, and participate in the evaluation.

Community organizations have traditionally been significantly underfunded compared with health systems, often operating with minimal resources and little in the way of analytic, information technology, and data collection capacity. To reduce the resource gap, the state allocated up to $100 million of the $650 million to enable the lead pilot entity and direct service providers to build their capacity and infrastructure in these areas.

A Final Word

"Health care has discovered community-based organizations and to some degree, community-based organizations are discovering health care, but there is a little bit of wariness still," Cindy Mann says. The contributors to this chapter propose strategies to reduce that wariness, introducing arguments and tools to demonstrate that emphasizing social determinants of health presents an opportunity for an ROI that may benefit multiple stakeholders while producing better health outcomes for their shared constituents.

They introduce new language that weaves together tenets of health care, the notion of community, and the potential of the economic argument. George Miller talks of "nonclinical prevention" and Cindy Mann describes "provider networks of community-based organizations," while in the previous chapter, Andrew Renda characterized social determinants as "clinical gaps in care." This new language suggests that progress has been made in the drive toward a Culture of Health and perhaps points to a new public narrative about what it means to be well. In time, as that "story" becomes embedded into the way we think about health and social services, we will have a better chance to more fully integrate whole-person strategies into the health care system.

Conclusion

As it draws together scholars, practitioners, and advocates across many disciplines, this volume of *Sharing Knowledge* underscores the need to shift core narratives and break down systemic barriers to resilience and equity. Recognizing the need to change mindsets—the assumptions and values that we bring to an issue—the contributors also point the ways toward what could be called *social determinants of health 2.0*.

Foundational articles published by Robert Wood Johnson Foundation (RWJF) leaders in 2002[1] and 2007[2] helped to identify contributing factors to premature death and mainstreamed the once-novel premise that social determinants have much more sway over health outcomes than health care. Those analyses attributed 40 percent of early mortality to behavioral patterns and only 10 percent to health care (the remainder is explained by genetic predisposition, social circumstances, and environmental exposures). By raising awareness of the true influences on health, RWJF helped to shift assumptions and inspired many sectors to act on the idea that health is mostly driven by what happens outside physicians' offices and hospitals. So accepted is this way of thinking now that it is hard to recall it was once a novel framework.

But that has left us with a lot to deconstruct. As we probe the origin story of the social determinants of health more deeply, we find ourselves asking: What is the cause behind the cause?[3] Talking about individual behavior can be a distraction if we don't also look at the social and economic conditions that limit healthy choices. If the crime or broken windows in a fractured community are all that draw our attention, we ignore the realities of disinvestment, racism, and the inequitable allocation of public services that broke those windows. Until we look at how waste plants are sited—and discover, as is reported elsewhere in this book, that in Houston all five city-owned landfills are located in Black neighborhoods—we won't know just why some populations are at higher risk for toxic exposure than others.

Conclusion In: *Community Resilience*. Edited by: Alonzo L. Plough, Oxford University Press (2021). © Robert Wood Johnson Foundation. DOI: 10.1093/oso/9780197559383.003.0022

A search for root causes then leads us to the ways in which American society marginalizes certain populations and especially to its enduring legacy of racial injustice. When a narrative is dominated by voices that lack diversity, when structures and systems close their doors to changemakers, the context in which to consider societal challenges remains narrow. At every level, we need to reconsider our frame. That means not only recognizing the importance of drawing in broader data sets but also reaching out to new sources to secure them. It means not only talking about being more inclusive but also bringing in new players as equal partners to redesign policy and practice.

Increasingly, RWJF is focusing its attention on those fundamentals. Beyond simply acknowledging the role of social determinants of health, we are conceptualizing them in ways that incorporate core equity issues and stretch our understanding of practices conducive to building a Culture of Health. Changing mindsets is key to this work because altering individual and societal assumptions creates a pathway to change: The stories we tell influence conversation and practice as they shift our view of what is normal and just.

We have seen that in our tobacco control work over the years—as smoking became much less socially acceptable, laws restricting it were easier to enact and enforce. Likewise, when inequity and racial injustice come to be seen as aberrant to a healthy society, we will be in a much stronger position to take aim at the entrenched structural forces that allow them to continue. To do that effectively, we need to become much more deliberate about how we consider the distribution and application of power—who has it, where it has been used and misused, and how it can be more equitably shared.

Building on these ideas, the fifth *Sharing Knowledge* conference, held in Jackson, Mississippi, in March 2020, was tightly focused on racial injustice, one of the nation's most durable and original forms of oppression. Drawing on what we have learned about systemic constraints on resilience and the imperative of inclusion, participants dug deep into some of the harshest truths embedded in the American story, wrongs that not only endanger the health of broad swaths of the population but also distort our democracy. Only by engaging fully in the struggle for equity and justice and combating racism in the many ways it is manifest can we advance toward a Culture of Health. After this conference took place, both the COVID-19 pandemic and many more brutal police homicides against Black people occurred. The need for deep social change, racial healing, and national and community resilience will be more important than ever going forward.

ACKNOWLEDGMENTS

The *Sharing Knowledge* conference involved the hard work of numerous individuals, both internal and external to the Robert Wood Johnson Foundation (RWJF). Tracy Costigan and Martina Todaro led the successful development of the conference in collaboration with Lisa Simpson and her staff at AcademyHealth. I also would like to thank the external steering committee, who helped develop the conference sessions.

Turning the fourth annual conference into this volume also required the vision and support of many. An editorial review group oversees the development of this series and provided careful commentary and suggestions. My colleagues in this group are Sandro Galea, Boston University; Sherry Glied, New York University; Anita Chandra, RAND Corporation; and Sarah Humphreville, Oxford University Press.

Special thanks to the team at RWJF who provided essential leadership and support throughout the development of this manuscript: Ketana Bhavsar, Ed Ghisu, Brian Quinn, and Kristin Silvani. Additional thanks to Rachel Bland and Jacquelynn Orr.

Finally, with guidance from RWJF staff, a team of talented writers crafted the manuscript, weaving together multiple data sources, including conference presentations and interviews, into cross-cutting chapters that reflect the conference objectives. Thank you for your excellent work Karyn Feiden, Mary B. Geisz, Margaret O. Kirk, and Mary Nakashian.

BIBLIOGRAPHY

Introduction

1. Costigan T. *What's the Formula for Community Resilience. Culture of Health Blog.* Robert Wood Johnson Foundation. August 1, 2016. www.rwjf.org/en/blog/2016/07/what_s_the_formulaf.html
2. Centers for Disease Control and Prevention. "COVID-19 in Racial and Ethnic Minorities." April 22, 2020. www.cdc.gov/coronavirus/2019-ncov/need-extra-precautions/racial-ethnic-minorities.html
3. Pew Research Center. "About Half of Lower-Income Americans Report Household Job or Wage Loss Due to COVID-19." *Social Trends,* April 21, 2020. www.pewsocialtrends.org/2020/04/21/about-half-of-lower-income-americans-report-household-job-or-wage-loss-due-to-covid-19/
4. Urban Institute. "The Covid Pandemic Is Straining Families' Ability to Afford Basic Needs." April 2020. www.rwjf.org/en/library/research/2020/04/covid-19-pandemic-was-already-straining-families-ability-to-afford-basic-needs-by-early-spring-with-low-income-and-his-panic-people-hardest-hit.html
5. Besser RA. "As Coronavirus Spreads, the Bill for Our Public Health Failures Is Due." *Washington Post,* March 5, 2020.

Chapter 1

1. Chetty R, Hendren N, Jones MR, et al. "Race and Economic Opportunity in the United States: An Intergenerational Perspective." *The Quarterly Journal of Economics,* 135(2), 711–718, 2020. https://doi.org/10.1093/qje/qjz042

Chapter 2

1. Graham C and Pettinato S. "Frustrated Achievers: Winners, Losers, and Subjective Well-Being in New Market Economies." *Journal of Development Studies,* 38(4), 100–140, 2002. https://doi.org/10.1080/00220380412331322431
2. Graham C, Laffan K, and Pinto S. "Well-Being in Metrics and Policy." *Science,* 362(6412), 287–288, October 2018. htttps://science.sciencemag.org/content/362/6412/287
3. Bureau of Labor Statistics. "The Employment Situation—March 2019," April 5, 2019. www.bls.gov/news.release/archives/empsit_04052019.pdf
4. Case A and Deaton A. "Rising Morbidity and Mortality in Midlife Among White Non-Hispanic Americans in the 21st Century." *Proceedings of the National Academy of Sciences of the United States of America (PNAS),* 112(49), 15078–15083, December 8, 2015. www.pnas.org/content/112/49/15078

5. Case A. "Fear and Despair: Consequences of Inequity." In *Knowledge to Action: Accelerating Progress in Health, Well-Being, and Equity.* Edited by Alonzo L Plough, 12–16. New York: Oxford University Press, 2017.

6. Xu J, Murphy SL, Kochaneck KD, et al. "Mortality in the United States, 2018." NCHS Data Brief No. 355, January 2020. www.cdc.gov/nchs/products/databriefs/db355.htm

7. O'Connor KJ and Graham C. "Longer, More Optimistic Lives: Historic Optimism and Life Expectancy in the United States." *Journal of Economic Behavior and Organization, 168,* 374–392, December 2019. www.sciencedirect.com/science/article/abs/pii/S016726811930325 7?via%3Dihub

8. Graham C and Pinto S. "Unequal Hopes and Lives in the U.S.A.: Optimism, Race, Place, and Premature Mortality." *Journal of Population Economics, 32*(2), 665–733, 2019. www.brookings.edu/wp-content/uploads/2017/06/working-paper-104-web-v2.pdf

9. Ibid.

10. Bloomberg Philanthropies. *Bloomberg Philanthropies Announces Mayors Challenge Winners Providence, Chicago, Houston, Philadelphia, and Santa Monica.* New York: Bloomberg Philanthropies, March 13, 2013. www.bloomberg.org/press/releases/bloomberg-philanthropies-announces-mayors-challenge-winners-providence-chicago-houston-philadelphia-and-santa-monica/

11. Office of Civic Wellbeing. *2019 Wellbeing Index Findings Preview.* Santa Monica, Calif.: Office of Civic Wellbeing, 2020. https://wellbeing.smgov.net/Media/Default/docs/wellbeing-preview-03092020.pdf

12. Flores W and Hernández A. "Health Accountability for Indigenous Populations: Confronting Power Through Adaptive Action Cycles." *IDS Bulletin: Transforming Development Knowledge, 49*(2), 19–34, 2018. https://bulletin.ids.ac.uk/index.php/idsbo/article/view/2963

13. Wahedi K, Flores W, Beiersmann C, et al. "Using Information Communication Technology to Identify Deficits in Rural Health Care: A Mixed-Methods Evaluation from Guatemala." *Global Health Action, 11*(1), Article 1455347, 2018. doi:10.1080/16549716.2018.1455347

14. Center for the Study of Equity and Governance in Health Systems (CEGSS), producer. *The Network of Community Defenders for the Right to Health.* Documentary. 2018. www.youtube.com/watch?v=g988GyYQ_1I&t=2s

15. Center for the Study of Equity and Governance in Health Systems (CEGSS), producer. *Citizens' Vigilance of Health Care Services and Accountability.* Documentary, 2015. www.youtube.com/watch?v=pJQlYlwQD4w&t=13s

16. Flores W. "How Can Evidence Bolster Citizen Action? Learning and Adapting for Accountable Public Health in Guatemala." Accountability Note 2. Accountability Research Center, 2018. http://accountabilityresearch.org/wp-content/uploads/2018/02/Accountability-Note2_English_2-22-18.pdf

17. Information about *Ring the Bell. One Million Men. One Million Promises* is available online. http://letsbreakthrough.org/nicp_mediacenter/one-million-men_one-million-promises-sir-patrick-stewart-made-his-promise-to-ring-the-bell/

Chapter 3

1. Gramlich J and Schaeffer K. "7 Facts About Guns in the U.S.," *Fact Tank,* October 22, 2019. www.pewresearch.org/fact-tank/2019/10/22/facts-about-guns-in-united-states/

2. "Small Arms Survey." Civilian Firearms Holdings, 2017. Accessed August 5, 2020. www.smallarmssurvey.org/fileadmin/docs/Weapons_and_Markets/Tools/Firearms_holdings/SAS-BP-Civilian-held-firearms-annexe.pdf

3. Information about the NRA is available at https://home.nra.org/about-the-nra/

4. Gramlich J. "What the Data Says About Gun Deaths in the U.S." *Fact Tank,* August 16, 2019. www.pewresearch.org/fact-tank/2019/08/16/what-the-data-says-about-gun-deaths-in-the-u-s/

5. Ibid.

6. Knopov A, Rothman EF, Cronin SW, et al. "The Role of Racial Residential Segregation in Black-White Disparities in Firearm Homicide at the State Level in the United States, 1991–2015." *JAMA, 111*(1), 62–75, February 2019. www.ncbi.nlm.nih.gov/pubmed/30129481

7. Ibid.

8. Ibid.
9. Ibid.
10. Gramlich and Schaeffer, "7 Facts About Guns in the U.S.".
11. Ibid.
12. Parker K, Horowitz JM, Igielnik R, et al. "America's Complex Relationship With Guns: An In-Depth Look at the Attitudes and Experiences of U.S. Adults." *Pew Research Center Social & Demographic Trends*, June 22, 2017. www.pewsocialtrends.org/2017/06/22/americas-complex-relationship-with-guns/
13. Bornstein DB and Davis WJ. "The Transportation Profession's Role in Improving Public Health." *Institute of Transportation Engineers Journal*, *84*(7), 19–24, July 1, 2014. www.researchgate.net/publication/264347123_The_Transportation_Profession%27s_Role_in_Improving_Public_Health/figures?lo=1
14. "Baltimore Homicides." *Baltimore Sun.* Interactive website. Accessed August 5, 2020. https://homicides.news.baltimoresun.com/?cause=shooting&range=2019
15. Siegel M, Sherman R, Li C, et al. "The Relationship Between Racial Residential Segregation and Black-White Disparities in Fatal Police Shootings at the City Level, 2013–2017." *Journal of the National Medical Association*, *111*(6), 580–587, December 2019. https://www.sciencedirect.com/science/article/abs/pii/S0027968419301300
16. Diez C, Kurland RP, Rothman EF, et al. "State Intimate Partner Violence-Related Firearm Laws and Intimate Partner Homicide Rates in the United States, 1991–2015." *Annals of Internal Medicine*, *167*(8), 536–543, 2017. https://annals.org/aim/fullarticle/2654047/state-intimate-partner-violence-related-firearm-laws-intimate-partner-homicide
17. Siegel M, Xuan Z, Ross CS, et al. "Easiness of Legal Access to Concealed Firearm Permits and Homicide Rates in the United States." *American Journal of Public Health*, *107*(12), November 8, 2017. https://ajph.aphapublications.org/doi/10.2105/AJPH.2017.304057
18. Siegel M, Pahn M, Xuan Z, et al. "The Impact of State Firearm Laws on Homicide and Suicide Deaths in the U.S., 1991–2016: A Panel Study." *Journal of General Internal Medicine*, 34, 2021–2028, March 28, 2019. https://link.springer.com/article/10.1007/s11606-019-04922-x
19. Information about the consortium is available at efsgv.org/consortium-risk-based-firearm-policy/about/
20. The toolkit is available at https://drive.google.com/file/d/1wSfzgeN4BJCQxBCZRB7LrMAXTN2F0t_o/view
21. The Educational Fund to Stop Gun Violence. "Data Behind Extreme Risk Laws: A Look at Connecticut's Risk-Warrant Law," July 2018. http://efsgv.org/wp-content/uploads/2018/07/Data-behind-Extreme-Risk-Laws_July-2018-5.pdf
22. Ibid.
23. The Educational Fund to Stop Gun Violence. "Guns, Public Health and Mental Illness: Summary of the Best Available Research Evidence," February 2018. http://efsgv.org/wp-content/uploads/2018/02/Guns-Public-Health-and-Mental-Illness-1.pdf
24. McLively M and Nieto B. "A Case Study in Hope: Lessons From Oakland's Remarkable Reduction in Gun Violence," April 23, 2019. https://lawcenter.giffords.org/a-case-study-in-hope-lessons-from-oaklands-remarkable-reduction-in-gun-violence/
25. Hohl BC, Kondo MC, Kajeepeta S, et al. "Creating Safe and Healthy Neighborhoods With Placed-Base Violence Interventions." *Health Affairs*, *38*(10), October 7, 2019. www.healthaffairs.org/doi/abs/10.1377/hlthaff.2019.00707?rfr_dat=cr_pub%3Dpubmed&url_ver=Z39.88-2003&rfr_id=ori%3Arid%3Acrossref.org&journalCode=hlthaff

Chapter 4

1. Budiman A, Tamir C, Mora L, and Noe-Bustamante L. "Facts on U.S. immigrants, 2018: Statistical portrait of the foreign-born population in the United States." *Hispanic Trends*. August 20, 2020. www.pewresearch.org/hispanic/2019/06/03/facts-on-u-s-immigrants/
2. Budiman A. "Key Findings About U.S. Immigrants." *Fact Tank*, August 20, 2020. www.pewresearch.org/fact-tank/2019/06/17/key-findings-about-u-s-immigrants/
3. U.S. Bureau of Labor Statistics. 2020. "Labor Force Characteristics of Foreign-born Workers Summary." www.bls.gov/news.release/forbrn.nr0.htm/labor-force-characteristics-of-foreign-born-workers-summary

4. Ibid.

5. National Immigration Forum. "Fact Sheet: E-Verify." 2018. https://immigrationforum.org/article/fact-sheet-e-verify/

6. U.S. Immigration and Customs Enforcement (ICE). "Delegation of Immigration Authority Section 287(g) Immigration and Nationality Act." Last update August 2, 2020. www.ice.gov/287g

7. Yoshikawa H, Chaudry A, Garcia SR, et al. *Approaches to Protect Children's Health and Human Services in an Era of Harsh Immigration Policy.* New York: New York University Institute of Human Development and Social Change, March 18, 2019. https://research.steinhardt.nyu.edu/scmsAdmin/media/users/ac190/IHDSC_Approaches_to_Protect_Childrens_Access_to_Health_and_Human_Services_in_an_Era_of_Harsh_Immigration_Policy.pdf

8. National Immigration Law Center. "State Laws Providing Access to Driver's Licenses or Cards, Regardless of Immigration Status." Last updated April 2020. www.nilc.org/wp-content/uploads/2015/11/drivers-license-access-table.pdf

9. Gelatt J, Bernstein H, and Koball H. "State Immigration Policy Resource." Urban Institute. 2017. www.urban.org/features/state-immigration-policy-resource

10. Gramlich J. "Far More Immigration Cases Are Being Prosecuted Criminally Under Trump Administration." *Fact Tank,* September 27, 2019. www.pewresearch.org/fact-tank/2019/09/27/far-more-immigration-cases-are-being-prosecuted-criminally-under-trump-administration/

11. Gelatt J, Koball H, Bernstein H, et al. "State Immigration Enforcement Policies: How They Impact Low-Income Households." Urban Institute. May 2017. www.nccp.org/publications/pdf/text_1182.pdf

12. Migration Policy Institute. "Unauthorized Immigrant Population Profiles." Accessed August 5, 2020. www.migrationpolicy.org/programs/us-immigration-policy-program-data-hub/unauthorized-immigrant-population-profiles

13. Martínez AD and Rhodes SD. "Introduction: Disentangling Language and the Social Determinants of Latinx Health in the United States." In *New and Emerging Issues in Latinx Health.* Edited by AD Martínez and SD Rhodes SD. Cham, Switzerland: Springer International, 2020. https://doi.org/10.1007/978-3-030-24043-1_1.

14. Capps R and Ruiz Soto AG. *A Profile of Houston's Immigrant Population in a Rapidly Changing Policy Landscape.* Washington, D.C.: Migration Policy Institute, September 2018. www.migrationpolicy.org/research/profile-houston-immigrant-population-changing-policy-landscape

15. Houston Immigration Legal Services Collaborative. *Humanitarian Action Plan: Recommendations for Coordinated Emergency Planning to Increase Immigrant Resilience.* Houston: Houston Immigration Legal Services Collaborative, March 2019. https://hap.houstonimmigration.org/assets/HAP_English.pdf

16. Capps and Ruiz Soto, *A Profile of Houston's Immigrant Population.*

17. Atkiss K, Vickery K, and Stys J. *Humanitarian Action Plan March 2019: Recommendations for Coordinated Emergency Planning to Increase Immigrant Resilience.* Houston: Houston Immigration Legal Services Collaborative, March 2019. www.hap.houstonimmigration.org/assets/HAP_English.pdf

18. Capps and Ruiz, 2018.

19. Fernandez M. "Texas Banned 'Sanctuary Cities.' Some Police Departments Didn't Get the Memo." *New York Times,* March 15, 2018. www.nytimes.com/2018/03/15/us/texas-sanctuary-sb4-immigration.html

20. "Counties Where ICE Arrests Concentrate." October 24, 2018. TRAC Immigration, Syracuse University. https://trac.syr.edu/immigration/reports/533/

21. Information on the Culture of Health Advancing Together (CHAT) program available at www.chattx.org

22. Theodore N. "After the Storm: Houston's Day Labor Markets in the Aftermath of Hurricane Harvey." Great Cities Institute, University of Illinois at Chicago. November 2017. https://greatcities.uic.edu/2017/11/21/after-the-storm-houstons-day-labor-markets-in-the-aftermath-of-hurricane-harvey/ and Wu B, Hamel L, Brodie M, et al. "Hurricane Harvey: The

Experience of Immigrants Living on the Texas Gulf Coast," Kaiser Family Foundation and Episcopal Health Foundation, March 20, 2018, www.kff.org/disparities-policy/report/hurricane-harvey-experiences-immigrants-texas-gulf-coast

23. See Note 22.

24. Anderson M and Lopez G. "Key Facts About Black Immigrants in the U.S." *Fact Tank,* January 24, 2018. www.pewresearch.org/fact-tank/2018/01/24/key-facts-about-Black-immigrants-in-the-u-s/

25. Lipscombe C, Morgan-Trostle J, and Zheng K. "The State of Black Immigrants." A report of the Black Alliance for Just Immigration and the New York University School of Law Immigrant Rights Clinic. Accessed August 5, 2020. www.stateofblackimmigrants.com/assets/sobi-fullreport-jan22.pdf

26. Ibid.

27. Ibid.

28. Ibid.

29. Partnership for a New American Economy. "Power of the Purse: How Sub-Saharan Africans Contribute to the U.S. Economy." January 2018. www.newamericaneconomy.org/wp-content/uploads/sites/2/2018/01/NAE_African_V6.pdf

30. U.S. Department of State. "Instructions for the 2021 Diversity Immigrant Visa Program (DV-2021)." Accessed August 5, 2020. www.travel.state.gov/content/dam/visas/Diversity-Visa/DV-Instructions-Translations/DV-2021-Instructions-Translations/DV-2021-%20Instructions-English.pdf

31. Ibid.

32. Ibid.

33. Klineberg SL. *The 2018 Kinder Houston Area Survey: Tracking Responses to Income Inequalities, Demographic Transformations, and Threatening Storms.* Houston: Rice/Kinder Institute for Urban Research, April 2018. https://scholarship.rice.edu/bitstream/handle/1911/105187/2018-report.pdf?sequence=1

Chapter 5

1. Lee MYH, "Does the United States Really Have 5 Percent of the World's Population and One Quarter of the World's Prisoners?" *Washington Post,* Fact Checker, April 30, 2015. www.washingtonpost.com/news/fact-checker/wp/2015/04/30/does-the-united-states-really-have-five-percent-of-worlds-population-and-one-quarter-of-the-worlds-prisoners/?noredirect=on&utm_term=.662ebeb01c4b

2. Widra E. "Incarceration Shortens Life Expectancy." *Prison Policy Initiative,* June 26, 2017. www.prisonpolicy.org/blog/2017/06/26/life_expectancy/

3. The Marshall Project. "A State-by-State Look at Coronavirus in Prisons." Updated July 30, 2020. www.themarshallproject.org/2020/05/01/a-state-by-state-look-at-coronavirus-in-prisons

4. Sawyer W and Wagner P. "Mass Incarceration: The Whole Pie 2019." *Prison Policy Initiative,* March 19, 2019. www.prisonpolicy.org/reports/pie2019.html

5. Gramlich J. "The Gap Between the Number of Blacks and Whites in Prison Is Shrinking." *Fact Tank,* April 30, 2019. www.pewresearch.org/fact-tank/2019/04/30/shrinking-gap-between-number-of-Blacks-and-Whites-in-prison/

6. Ibid.

7. Sawyer W and Wagner P. "Mass Incarceration: The Whole Pie 2020." *Prison Policy Initiative,* March 24, 2020. www.prisonpolicy.org/reports/pie2020.html

8. Ibid.

9. Waters M. "How Prisons Are Poisoning Their Inmates: Hundreds of U.S. Prisons and ICE Detention Centers Are Built on Toxic Sites, and People Inside Are Getting Sick." *The Outline—Power,* July 23, 2018. https://theoutline.com/post/5410/toxic-prisons-fayette-tacoma-contaminated?zd=1&zi=zl6u374o

10. Bernd C, Loftus-Farren Z, and Mitra MN. "America's Toxic Prisons: The Environmental Injustices of Mass Incarceration." *Earth Island Journal,* Summer 2017. http://earthisland.org/journal/americas-toxic-prisons/

11. Abolitionist Law Center. *No Escape: Exposure to Toxic Coal Waste at State Correctional Institution Fayette.* Pittsburgh: Abolitionist Law Center, 2014. https://abolitionistlawcenter. org/wp-content/uploads/2014/09/no-escape-3-3mb.pdf

12. Omorogieva W. *Prison Preparedness and Legal Obligations to Protect Prisoners During Natural Disasters.* New York: Sabin Center for Climate Change Law, Columbia Law School, May 2018. http://columbiaclimatelaw.com/files/2018/05/Omorogieva-2018-05-Prison-Preparedness-and-Legal-Obligations.pdf

13. Annie E. Casey Foundation. *Children of Incarcerated Parents, a Shared Sentence: The Devastating Toll of Parental Incarceration on Kids, Families and Communities.* Baltimore: Annie E. Casey Foundation, April 18, 2016. www.aecf.org/resources/a-shared-sentence?gclid =Cj0KCQiArdLvBRCrARIsAGhB_syVkD2N0qUbHv3NlErrkAqaB1xSMUB4zMwZ_ 6Cqfh25FRCpwfqJhHQaAhIQEALw_wcB/#key-takeaway

14. Wakefield S and Wildeman C. "Paternal Incarceration and Infant Mortality," In *Children of the Prison Boom: Mass Incarceration and the Future of American Inequality,* 97–112. New York: Oxford University Press, 2013. www.oxfordscholarship.com/view/10.1093/ acprof:oso/9780199989225.001.0001/acprof-9780199989225-chapter-5

15. Johnson RC and Raphael S. "The Effects of Male Incarceration Dynamics on Acquired Immune Deficiency Syndrome Infection Rates Among African American Women and Men." *Journal of Law and Economics,* 52(2), 251–293, 2009. https://gspp.berkeley.edu/assets/ uploads/research/pdf/P48.pdf

16. Enns PK, Youngmin Y, Comfort M, et al. "What Percentage of Americans Have Ever Had a Family Member Incarcerated?: Evidence From the Family History of Incarceration Survey (FamHIS)." *Socius,* 5, 1–45. https://journals.sagepub.com/doi/pdf/10.1177/ 2378023119829332

17. Elderbroom B, Bennett L, Gong S, et al. "Every Second: The Impact of the Incarceration Crisis on America's Families." FWD.us, 2018. https://everysecond.fwd.us/downloads/ EverySecond.fwd.us.pdf

18. Venters H. *Life and Death in Rikers Island.* Baltimore: Johns Hopkins University Press, 2019, 3.

19. Ibid.

20. Ibid.

21. Ulrich RS. "View Through a Window May Influence Recovery From Surgery." *Science,* 224(4647), 420–421, May 1984. www.researchgate.net/publication/17043718_View_ Through_a_Window_May_Influence_Recovery_from_Surgery

22. Haney C. "The Psychological Effects of Solitary Confinement: A Systematic Critique." *Crime and Justice,* 47(1), 365–416, March 9, 2018. www.journals.uchicago.edu/doi/full/10.1086/ 696041

23. Cheek F and Miller MDS. "Reducing Staff and Inmate Stress." *Corrections Today,* 44(5), 72– 76, 1982. www.ncjrs.gov/App/Publications/abstract.aspx?ID=85591

24. Parker JR. *Florida Mortality Study: Florida Law Enforcement and Corrections Officers Compared to Florida General Population.* Brevard County, FL: Office of the Sheriff, October 17, 2011. http://www.floridastatefop.org/pdf_files/floridamortalitystudy.pdf

25. Lerman AE. *Officer Health and Wellness: Results From the California Correctional Officer Survey.* Berkeley, Calif.: University of California, Berkeley, 2017.

26. Samson L. "Can the Architecture of a Prison Contribute to the Rehabilitation of Its Inmates?" *Design Indaba,* April 29, 2019. www.designindaba.com/articles/creative-work/ can-architecture-prison-contribute-rehabilitation-its-inmates

27. Ibid.

Chapter 6

1. Matin N, Forrester J, and Ensor J. "What Is Equitable Resilience?" *World Development,* 109, 197–205, September 2018. doi.org/10.1016/j.worlddev.2018.04.020

2. Centers for Disease Control and Prevention. "U.S. Opioid Prescribing Rate Maps, Key Highlights." Last updated March 5, 2020. www.cdc.gov/drugoverdose/maps/rxrate-maps. html

3. Centers for Disease Control and Prevention, National Center for Injury Prevention and Control, U.S. Department of Health and Human Services. "Annual Surveillance Report of Drug-Related Risks and Outcomes: United States, 2019." Executive Summary, p. 7. www.cdc.gov/drugoverdose/pdf/pubs/2019-cdc-drug-surveillance-report.pdf

4. Goodnough A, Katz J, and Sanger-Katz M. "Drug Overdose Deaths Drop in U.S. for First Time Since 1990." *New York Times,* July 17, 2019. www.nytimes.com/interactive/2019/07/17/upshot/drug-overdose-deaths-fall.html

5. "Drugmaker's Opioid Settlement Offer Gains Ground With States." *Claims Journal,* February 26, 2020. www.claimsjournal.com/news/national/2020/02/26/295692.htm

6. "Medications for Opioid Use Disorder Save Lives." A consensus study report by the National Academies of Sciences, Engineering, and Medicine. March 2019. Highlights. www.Nationalacademies.org/OUDtreatment

7. "Confronting Our Nation's Opioid Crisis." A report of the Aspen Health Strategy Group, with funding provided by Robert Wood Johnson Foundation, the Laura and John Arnold Foundation, and the Laurie M. Tisch Illumination Fund. January 11, 2018. www.aspeninstitute.org/publications/confronting-our-nations-opioid-crisis/

8. Centers for Disease Control and Prevention. "Understanding the Epidemic: The Three Waves of Opioid Overdose Deaths." www.cdc.gov/drugoverdose/epidemic/index.html

9. Katz J and Sanger-Katz M. "The Numbers Are So Staggering. Overdose Deaths Set a Record Last Year," *New York Times,* November 29, 2018. www.nytimes.com/interactive/2018/11/29/upshot/fentanyl-drug-overdose-deaths.html

10. National Institute on Drug Abuse. "Trends and Statistics: Overdose Death Rates," March 10, 2020. www.drugabuse.gov/drug-topics/trends-statistics/overdose-death-rates

11. Centers for Disease Control and Prevention. CDC WONDER: Wide-Ranging Online Data for Epidemiologic Research (WONDER), 2017. http://wonder.cdc.gov

12. The individuals named in this paragraph are five real faces of the opioid crisis; their stories were reported in the media.

13. Giroir BP. "The Opioid Epidemic and Emerging Public Health Policy Priorities." Office of the Assistant Secretary for Health, February 13, 2019. www.ama-assn.org/system/files/2019-02/19-nac-opioid-epidemic-presentation_0.pdf

14. Maiolo D. "State Senators Seek to Expand Routt County Addiction Treatment Program." *Steamboard Pilot & Today,* February 28, 2019. www.steamboatpilot.com/news/state-senators-seek-to-expand-routt-county-addiction-treatment-program/

15. Ibid.

16. Ibid.

17. Wagner P. "Incarceration Is Not an Equal Opportunity Punishment." *Prison Policy Initiative,* August 28, 2012. www.prisonpolicy.org/articles/notequal.html

18. Vestal C. "New Momentum for Addiction Treatment Behind Bars." *Stateline,* April 4, 2018. www.pewtrusts.org/en/research-and-analysis/blogs/stateline/2018/04/04/new-momentum-for-addiction-treatment-behind-bars

19. Bronson J, Stroop J, Zimmer S, et al. "Drug Use, Dependence, and Abuse Among State Prisoners and Jail Inmates, 2007–2009." U.S. Department of Justice, p. 1, June 2017. www.bjs.gov/content/pub/pdf/dudaspji0709.pdf

20. National Institute on Drug Abuse. "Drug Facts, Criminal Justice." June 2019. www.drugabuse.gov/publications/drugfacts/criminal-justice

21. Vaughn E. "Opioid Addiction in Jails: An Anthropologist's Perspective." *Shots: Health News from National Public Radio,* November 12, 2019. www.npr.org/sections/health-shots/2019/11/12/777586941/opioid-addiction-in-jails-an-anthropologists-perspective

22. Ibid.

23. Ibid.

24. Ranapurwala SI, Shanahan ME, Alexandridis AA, et al. "Opioid Overdose Mortality Among Former North Carolina Inmates: 2000–2015." *American Journal of Public Health, 108*(9), 1207–1213, September 2018. www.ncbi.nlm.nih.gov/pmc/articles/PMC6085027/

25. Gelb A and Velazquez T. "The Changing State of Recidivism: Fewer People Going Back to Prison." Pew Charitable Trusts, August 1, 2018. www.pewtrusts.org/en/research-and-analysis/articles/2018/08/01/the-changing-state-of-recidivism-fewer-people-going-back-to-prison

26. Ibid.
27. Volkow N. "The Importance of Treating Opioid Use Disorder in the Justice System." National Institute on Drug Abuse, July 24, 2019. www.drugabuse.gov/about-nida/noras-blog/2019/07/importance-treating-opioid-use-disorder-in-justice-system
28. "Case Study: Middlesex County, MA: A County Participates in a Legislatively-Driven MAT Expansion." Unpublished. Provided by Elizabeth Connolly, Pew Charitable Trusts.
29. American Medical Association, The Colorado Medical Society, and Manatt Health. "Spotlight on Colorado: Best Practices and Next Steps in the Opioid Epidemic." January 2019. www.end-opioid-epidemic.org/wp-content/uploads/2019/01/AMA-Paper-Spotlight-on-Colorado-January-2019_FOR-WEB.pdf
30. City and County of Denver, Department of Public Health and Environment. "Opioid Response Strategic Plan 2019–2023." www.denvergov.org/content/dam/denvergov/Portals/771/documents/CH/Substance%20Misuse/DDPHE_OpioidResponseStrategicPlan.pdf
31. Bachrach D, Frohlich J, Cantrall C, et al. "Communities in Crisis." Rural Health and Well-Being in America, a RWJF Collection, published by Manatt Health, October 27, 2017. www.rwjf.org/en/library/research/2017/10/communities-in-crisis--local-responses-to-behavioral-health-challenges.html
32. American Academy of Family Physicians. "More Opioids Being Prescribed in Rural America," January 28, 2019. www.aafp.org/news/health-of-the-public/20190128ruralopioids.html
33. Ibid.
34. Gale J, Janis J, Coburn A, et al. "Behavioral Health in Rural America: Challenges and Opportunities." Maine Rural Health Research Center, University of Southern Maine, October 2019. www.rupri.org/wp-content/uploads/Behavioral-Health-in-Rural-America-Challenges-and-Opportunities.pdf
35. Ibid.
36. Ibid.
37. "Rural Leadership, Rural Health: What We're Learning." Robert Wood Johnson Foundation, Rural Health and Well-Being in America, July 1, 2019. www.rwjf.org/en/library/research/2019/06/rural-leadership--rural-health.html
38. National Institute on Drug Abuse. "Maine Opioid Summary: Opioid-Involved Overdose Deaths." March 2019. www.drugabuse.gov/drug-topics/opioids/opioid-summaries-by-state/maine-opioid-involved-deaths-related-harms
39. Project Lazarus. Home page. www.projectlazarus.org
40. Rural Health Information Hub. "Midcoast Maine Prescription Opioid Reduction Program." www.ruralhealthinfo.org/project-examples/893
41. Rural Health Information Hub. "Keepin' It REAL Rural." www.ruralhealthinfo.org/project-examples/872
42. Ibid.
43. Ibid.
44. Ibid.
45. Ibid.
46. Ibid.
47. Ibid.
48. State of Vermont. "Hub and Spoke, Vermont's Opioid Use Disorder Treatment System, a Blueprint for Health." www.blueprintforhealth.vermont.gov/about-blueprint/hub-and-spoke
49. Ibid.
50. Manatt, Phelps & Phillips, LLP. "Medicaid's Role in Fighting the Opioid Epidemic. Briefing Series: Key Medicaid Issues for New State Policymakers," Issue 6, February 2019. Rural Health and Well-Being in America, a RWJF Collection. www.rwjf.org/en/library/research/2019/02/medicaid-s-role-in-fighting-the-opioid-epidemic.html
51. Ibid.
52. Ibid.
53. Vestal C. "As the Opioid Crisis Peaks, Meth and Cocaine Deaths Explode." *Stateline*, May 13, 2019. www.pewtrusts.org/en/research-and-analysis/blogs/stateline/2019/05/13/as-the-opioid-crisis-peaks-meth-and-cocaine-deaths-explode

54. Thistle S. "Despite Efforts to Stem Epidemic, Maine Overdose Deaths Appear to Be on the Rise Again After 1-Year Dip." *Press Herald*, January 23, 2019. www.pressherald.com/2020/01/23/new-report-shows-maine-drug-overdose-deaths-increasing-in-2019/

Chapter 7

1. Felitti VJ, Anda RF, Nordenberg D, et al. "Relationship of Childhood Abuse and Household Dysfunction to Many of the Leading Causes of Death in Adults: The Adverse Childhood Experiences (ACE) Study." *American Journal of Preventive Medicine, 14*(4), 245–258, 1998. www.ajpmonline.org/article/S0749-3797(98)00017-8/abstract
2. Burke Harris N. *The Deepest Well: Healing the Long-Term Effects of Childhood Adversity.* Boston: Houghton Mifflin Harcourt, 2018.
3. California Health and Human Service Agency. "Office of the California Surgeon General," 2019. www.chhs.ca.gov/office-of-the-california-surgeon-general/
4. Center for Youth Wellness. *An Unhealthy Dose of Stress: The Impact of Adverse Childhood Experiences and Toxic Stress on Childhood Health and Development.* San Francisco: Center for Youth Wellness, 2013. https://drive.google.com/file/d/1RD50llP2dimEdV3zn0eGrgtCi2TWfakH/view
5. National Pediatric Practice Community on Adverse Childhood Experiences (NPPCACES). Home page. https://nppcaces.org/
6. Teicher MH, Samson JA, Anderson CM, et al. "The Effects of Childhood Maltreatment on Brain Structure, Function and Connectivity." *Nature Reviews Neuroscience, 17*(10), 652–666, 2016. www.ncbi.nlm.nih.gov/pubmed/27640984
7. Teicher MH and Samson JA. "Annual Research Review: Enduring Neurobiological Effects of Childhood Abuse and Neglect." *Journal of Child Psychology and Psychiatry, 57*(3), 241–266, 2016. www.ncbi.nlm.nih.gov/pubmed/26831814
8. Heim CM, Mayberg HS, Mletzko T, et al. "Decreased Cortical Representation of Genital Somatosensory Field After Childhood Sexual Abuse." *American Journal of Psychiatry, 170*(6), 616–623, 2013. www.ncbi.nlm.nih.gov/pubmed/23732967
9. Teicher MH, Anderson CM, Ohashi K, et al. "Differential Effects of Childhood Neglect and Abuse During Sensitive Exposure Periods on Male and Female Hippocampus." *NeuroImage, 169*, 443–452, 2018. www.ncbi.nlm.nih.gov/pubmed/29288867
10. Zhu J, Lowen SB, Anderson CM, et al. "Association of Prepubertal and Postpubertal Exposure to Childhood Maltreatment With Adult Amygdala Function." *JAMA Psychiatry, 76*(8), 843–853, 2019. https://jamanetwork.com/journals/jamapsychiatry/article-abstract/2737199
11. Ibid.
12. Ohashi K, Anderson CM, Bolger EA, et al. "Childhood Maltreatment Is Associated With Alteration in Global Network Fiber-Tract Architecture Independent of History of Depression and Anxiety." *NeuroImage, 150*, 50–59, 2017. www.ncbi.nlm.nih.gov/pubmed/28213111
13. Ohashi K, Anderson CM, Bolger EA, et al. "Susceptibility or Resilience to Maltreatment Can Be Explained by Specific Differences in Brain Network Architecture." *Biological Psychiatry, 85*(8), 690–702, 2019. www.ncbi.nlm.nih.gov/pubmed/30528381
14. Morris AS, Hays-Grudo J, Treat A., et al. *Assessing Resilience Using the Protective and Compensatory Experiences Survey (PACES).* Poster, 2015. www.acesandpaces.com/uploads/6/4/3/1/64312853/srcd_2015_paces_poster_final.pdf
15. Hays-Grudo J and Morris AS. *Adverse and Protective Childhood Experiences: A Developmental Perspective.* Washington: American Psychological Association, 2020. www.apa.org/pubs/books/adverse-protective-childhood-experiences
16. Hays-Grudo J. *Adversity and Resilience Science: Journal of Research and Practice.* Home page. Springer, 2020. www.springer.com/journal/42844
17. Diaz A, Simatov E, and Rickert VI. "Effect of Abuse on Health: Results of a National Survey." *Archives of Pediatric Adolescent Medicine, 156*(8), 811–817, 2002. https://jamanetwork.com/journals/jamapediatrics/fullarticle/203769
18. Widom CS and Maxfield MG. "An Update of the 'Cycle of Violence.'" *National Institute of Justice: Research in Brief*, February 2001. www.ncjrs.gov/pdffiles1/nij/184894.pdf.

19. Baglivio MT, Epps N, Swartz K, et al. "The Prevalence of Adverse Childhood Experiences (ACE) in the Lives of Juvenile Offenders." *Journal of Juvenile Justice*, 3(2), 1–17, 2014. www. prisonpolicy.org/scans/Prevalence_of_ACE.pdf

20. Cronholm PF, Forke CM, Wade R, et al. "Adverse Childhood Experiences: Expanding the Concept of Adversity." *American Journal of Preventive Medicine*, 49(3), 354–361, 2015. www. ncbi.nlm.nih.gov/pubmed/26296440

21. Epstein R, Blake JJ, and González T. *Girlhood Interrupted: The Erasure of Black Girls' Childhood.* Washington: Center for Poverty and Inequality, Georgetown University Law Center, 2017. www.law.georgetown.edu/poverty-inequality-center/wp-content/uploads/sites/14/2017/08/girlhood-interrupted.pdf

22. Crenshaw KW, Ocen P, and Nanda J. *Black Girls Matter: Pushed Out, Overpoliced and Underprotected.* New York: African American Policy Forum and Center for Intersectionality and Social Policy Studies, 2015. www.atlanticphilanthropies.org/wp-content/uploads/2015/09/BlackGirlsMatter_Report.pdf

23. Gregory A and Evans KR. *The Starts and Stumbles of Restorative Justice in Education: Where Do We Go From Here?* Boulder, Colo.: National Education Policy Center, 2020. https://nepc.colorado.edu/publication/restorative-justice

Spotlight

1. Womble A. *Everybody Hurts: The State of Mental Health in America.* New York: Crisis Text Line, 2020. www.crisistextline.org/mental-health/everybody-hurts-the-state-of-mental-health-in-america/

2. Thompson LK, Michael KD, Runkle J, et al. "Crisis Text Line Use Following the Release of Netflix Series *13 Reasons Why* Season 1: Time-Series Analysis of Help-Seeking Behavior in Youth." *Preventive Medicine Reports*, 14, February 2019. www.ncbi.nlm.nih.gov/pubmed/30828539

3. Sugg MM, Michael KD, Stevens SS, et al. "Crisis Text Patterns in Youth Following the Release of *13 Reasons Why* Season 2 and Celebrity Suicides: A Case Study of Summer 2018." *Preventive Medicine Reports*, October 2019. www.sciencedirect.com/science/article/pii/S2211335519301706

4. Sugg MM, Dixon PG, and Runkle JD. "Crisis Support-Seeking Behavior and Temperature in the United States: Is There an Association in Young Adults and Adolescents?" *Science of the Total Environment*, 669, 400–411, 2019. www.sciencedirect.com/science/article/pii/S0048969719309465

5. Thompson LK, Sugg MM, and Runkle JR. "Adolescents in Crisis: A Geographic Exploration of Help-Seeking Behavior Using Data from Crisis Text Line." *Social Science & Medicine*, 215, 69–70, 2018. www.ncbi.nlm.nih.gov/pubmed/30216891

Chapter 8

1. Dubay L. "The State of the Nation's Housing 2019." Presentation slide at *Sharing Knowledge* 2019. Joint Center for Housing Studies, Harvard University. www.jchs.harvard.edu/state-nations-housing-2019

2. "U.S. Census Bureau, Decennial Censuses of Population and Housing and American Communities Survey Five-Year Estimates, Based on Authors Calculations." Slides presented by Smedley at *Sharing Knowledge* 2019.

3. Ibid.

4. "2005–08 Office of Epidemiology/Policy and Planning, Baltimore City Department of Planning." Slides presented by Smedley at *Sharing Knowledge* 2019.

5. Galster GC. "The Mechanism(s) of Neighbourhood Effects: Theory, Evidence, and Policy Implications." *Neighbourhood Effects Research: New Perspectives*, Spring 2012. http://archive.clas.wayne.edu/Multimedia/DUSP/files/G.Galster/St_AndrewsSeminar-Mechanisms_of_neigh_effects-Galster_2-23-10.pdf

6. Reyes-Nash L. "Health Is Housing." Poster presentation, at *Sharing Knowledge* conference, Houston, 2019. Chicago housing data from the University of Illinois Health Hospital and Clinics, 2016.

7. Byrne T and Miller DP. "Does the Value of Housing Assistance Impact Health Outcomes?" Policies for Action, Robert Wood Johnson Foundation. www.policiesforaction.org/project/does-value-housing-assistance-impact-health-outcomes

8. Center for Budget and Policy Priorities. "Three Out of Four Low-Income At-Risk Renters Do Not Receive Federal Rental Assistance." Chart developed from HUD custom tabulations of the 2015 American Housing Survey; 2016 HUD administrative data; FY2016 McKinney-Vento Permanent Supportive Housing bed counts; 2015–2016 Housing Opportunities for Persons with AIDS grantee performance profiles; and the USDA FY2016 Multi-Family Fair Housing Occupancy Report. http://apps.cbpp.org/shareables_housing_unmet/chart.html

9. Cunningham MK, Galvez MM, Aranda C., et al. "A Pilot Study of Landlord Acceptance of Housing Choice Vouchers." Urban Institute, September 2018. www.huduser.gov/portal/pilot-study-landlord-acceptance-hcv.html

10. Cohen-Cline H and Vartanian K. "Exploring a Targeted Housing Voucher Strategy." Providence Portland Medical Center. www.policiesforaction.org/project/exploring-targeted-housing-voucher-strategy

11. Ahrentzen S. and Dearborn L. "Shaping Healthier Housing for Low-Income and Vulnerable Populations." Policies for Action, Robert Wood Johnson Foundation. www.policiesforaction.org/project/shaping-healthier-housing-low-income-and-vulnerable-populations

12. STV AECOM PNA—A Joint Venture. "Physical Needs Assessment 2017." Report prepared for New York City Housing Authority. March 25, 2018. www1.nyc.gov/assets/nycha/downloads/pdf/PNA%202017.pdf.

13. Glied S. "NYU Wagner Graduate School of Public Service." Policies for Action, Robert Wood Johnson Foundation. www.policiesforaction.org/hub/new-york-university-wagner-graduate-school-public-service

14. Ibid.

15. Dragan KL, Ellen IG, and Glied SA. "Gentrification and the Health of Low-Income Children in New York City." *Health Affairs,* 38(9), 2019. https://www.healthaffairs.org/doi/full/10.1377/hlthaff.2018.05422

16. Reyes-Nash L. "Health Is Housing." Poster presentation, at *Sharing Knowledge* conference, Houston, 2018. Los Angeles housing data from RAND, Evaluation of Housing for Health Permanent Supportive Housing Program, 2017.

17. Moore Q, Richards A, and Kulesza C. "Third Ward Comprehensive Needs Assessment Data Report." October 2019. https://www.bakerinstitute.org/media/files/files/21d6e093/chb-pub-thirdward-102119.pdf

18. Katz LF. "Moving to Opportunity for Fair Housing Demonstration Program: Final Impacts Evaluation." http://www.nber.org/mtopublic/final.htm

19. Perry A, Rothwell J, and Harshbarger D. "The Devaluation of Assets in Black Neighborhoods: The Case of Residential Property." Metropolitan Policy Program at Brookings Institution. November 2018. https://www.brookings.edu/wp-content/uploads/2018/11/2018.11_Brookings-Metro_Devaluation-Assets-Black-Neighborhoods_final.pdf

20. Choi A, Herbert K, Winslow O, et al. "Long Island Divided." *Newsday,* November 17, 2019.https://projects.newsday.com/long-island/real-estate-agents-investigation/

21. Perry A. *Know Your Price: Valuing Black Lives and Property in America's Black Cities.* Washington, DC: Brookings Institution Press, May 2020. https://www.brookings.edu/book/know-your-price/

22. Scally CP, Waxman E, Gourevitch R, et al. "Emerging Strategies for Integrating Health and Housing". Urban Institute, July 20, 2017. https://www.urban.org/research/publication/emerging-strategies-integrating-health-and-housing

Chapter 9

1. Lindau ST, Makelarski J, Abramsohn E, et al. "CommunityRx: A Population Health Improvement Innovation That Connects Clinics to Communities." *Health Affairs*, 35(11), 2020–2029, 2016. www.ncbi.nlm.nih.gov/pubmed/27834242
2. The THRIVE website at https://thrivegreatlakesbay.org provides extensive information about THRIVE history, framework, and current activities.
3. Homer J. "Reference Guide for the ReThink Health Dynamics Simulation Model: A Tool for Regional Health System Transformation, Model Version 3v." Prepared for the Fannie. E. Rippel Foundation, Morristown, NJ, November 2018, www.rethinkhealth.org/wp-content/uploads/2019/09/ReThink-Health-Dynamics-Reference-Guide-v3v-Nov-2018-1.pdf

Chapter 10

1. "Building and Measuring Community Resilience: Actions for Communities and the Gulf Research Program." A consensus study report of the National Academies of Sciences, Engineering, Medicine. 2019. www.nap.edu/catalog/25383/building-and-measuring-community-resilience-actions-for-communities-and-the
2. Chandra A, Acosta J, Stern S, et al. "Building Community Resilience to Disasters: A Way Forward to Enhance National Health Security." Sponsored by the U.S. Department of Health and Human Services, research conducted in RAND Health, a division of the RAND Corporation. 2011. www.rand.org/content/dam/rand/pubs/technical_reports/2011/RAND_TR915.pdf
3. 218 Ibid.
4. "Disaster Resilience: A National Imperative." A consensus study report of the National Academies of Sciences, Engineering, Medicine. 2012. www.nap.edu/catalog/13457/disaster-resilience-a-national-imperative
5. Ibid.
6. Ibid.
7. "ResilientAmerica Roundtable, Community Pilot Program." National Academies of Sciences, Engineering, Medicine. www.nationalacademies.org/our-work/resilient-america-community-pilot-program
8. Cedar Rapids/Linn County, Iowa, ResilientAmerica partnership. www.nationalacademies.org/our-work/cedar-rapidslinn-county-ia-pilot-community
9. Charleston, South Carolina, ResilientAmerica partnership. www.nationalacademies.org/our-work/charleston-sc-pilot-community
10. Central Puget Sound Region, Washington, ResilientAmerica partnership. www.nationalacademies.org/our-work/central-puget-sound-region-wa-pilot-community
11. State Impact Oklahoma. "In Tulsa, a National Blueprint for Managing Floods as Cities Grow and Climate Changes." National Public Radio, November 2017. stateimpact.npr.org/oklahoma/2017/11/02/in-tulsa-a-national-blueprint-for-managing-floods-as-cities-grow-and-climate-changes/
12. Tulsa, Oklahoma, ResilientAmerica partnership. www.nationalacademies.org/our-work/tulsa-ok-pilot-community
13. "About the Gulf Research Program. National Academies of Sciences, Engineering, Medicine. www.nationalacademies.org/gulf/about/index.html
14. "After Katrina—Combating Mental Illness." Program Results Report. Robert Wood Johnson Foundation, April 2011. www.rwjf.org/en/library/research/2011/04/after-katrina.html
15. Thriving Community Grant Awards. "Community Resilience Learning Collaborative and Research Network." 2017. Total grant awarded $2,522,193. www.nationalacademies.org/gulf/grants/awards/thriving-communities/index.htm#thriving4
16. According to Springgate, the C-LEARN model reflects the work of the Los Angeles-based Community Partners in Care study led by Kenneth Wells and former mentor Loretta Jones and echoes elements of the 2010–2013 work of the Los Angeles County Community Disaster Resilience Initiative, headed by then Public Health Commissioner Alonzo Plough before he joined RWJF. For more on the work of Wells and Jones, see "Community Partners in Care,"

UCLA Semel Institute, Health Services and Society. https://hss.semel.ucla.edu/portfolio/community-partners-in-care/Community, Partners in Care study led by Kenneth Wells and Loretta Jones.

17. Pollack MJ, Wennerstrom A, True G, et al. "Preparedness and Community Resilience in Disaster-Prone Areas: Cross-Sectoral Collaborations in South Louisiana, 2018." *American Journal of Public Health, Open-Themed Research,* 109(Supplement 4), 2019. https://ajph.aphapublications.org/doi/10.2105/AJPH.2019.305152

18. C-Learn.org. "Our Work." www.c-learn.org/about

19. Ibid.

20. Ibid.

21. C-LEARN—Community Resilience Learning Collaborative and Research Network. "Phase One: Key Information Interviews." www.c-learn.org/phase-one

22. Ibid.

23. Ibid.

24. C-LEARN—Community Resilience Learning Collaborative and Research Network. "Phase Two: Interventions." www.c-learn.org/phase-two

25. Springgate BF, Arevian AC, Wennerstrom A, et al. "Community Resilience Learning Collaborative and Research Network (C-LEARN): Study Protocol With Participatory Planning for a Randomized, Comparative Effectiveness Trial." *International Journal of Environmental Research and Public Health,* 15(8), August 7, 2018. https://read.qxmd.com/read/30720791/community-resilience-learning-collaborative-and-research-network-c-learn-study-protocol-with-participatory-planning-for-a-randomized-comparative-effectiveness-trial

26. del Pino HE, Jones L, Forge N, et al. "Integrating Community Expertise Into the Academy: South Los Angeles' Community-Academic Model for Partnered Research." *Progress in Community Health Partnerships: Research, Education, and Action,* 10(2), 329–338, 2016. www.ncbi.nlm.nih.gov/pmc/articles/PMC5201428/

27. Davis R, Pinderhighes H, and Williams M. "Adverse Community Experiences and Resilience: A Framework for Addressing and Preventing Community Trauma." Prevention Institute. February 2016. https://www.preventioninstitute.org/publications/adverse-community-experiences-and-resilience-framework-addressing-and-preventing

28. Although the acronym is the same, the Prevention Institute's THRIVE initiative is unrelated to the THRIVE initiative in Central Michigan described in the previous chapter.

29. "THRIVE: Tool for Health and Resilience in Vulnerable Environments." Prevention Institute. www.preventioninstitute.org/tools/thrive-tool-health-resilience-vulnerable-environments

30. Ibid.

31. Ibid.

Spotlight

1. "Inland from the Coast: A Multi-Scalar Approach to Regional Climate Change Responses," presentation by Traci L. Birch, PhD, AICP, at the RWJF "Knowledge to Action" Conference in Houston, Texas, March 2019.

2. Robert Wood Johnson Foundation, "National Academies' Gulf Research Program and RWJF Award $10.8 million to Build Health, Resilient Coast Communities," press release, July 18, 2017. www.rwjf.org/en/library/articles-and-news/2017/07/national-academies-gulf-research-program-and-rwjf-award-10-8-million-to-build-healthy-resilient-coastal-communities.html

Chapter 11

1. Flavelle C. "In Houston, a Rash of Storms Tests the Limits of Coping with Climate Change." *The New York Times,* October 2, 2019. www.nytimes.com/2019/10/02/climate/hurricane-adaptation-houston.html

2. Population Report, January 2019, Harris County, Texas. https://budget.harriscountytx.gov/doc/Budget/fy2020/approved_budget/FY20_Population_Report.pdf

3. World Population Review, Houston, Texas. www.worldpopulationreview.com/us-cities/houston-population/
4. Ibid.
5. Ibid.
6. Trickey E. "The Health App That Beat Hurricane Harvey," *Politico*, January 18, 2018. www.politico.com/magazine/story/2018/01/18/what-works-health-app-harvey-216479
7. Texas Flood Registry (formerly the Hurricane Harvey Registry). https://floodregistry.rice.edu/
8. Harris County Public Health. "One Year After Harvey." YouTube video.www.youtube.com/playlist?list=PLOBJgqWGHBJGS6Uor9-Or5BUxxwzdvzp2
9. Harris County Public Health. "One Year After Harvey—Patrick & Xiomi." YouTube video. August 30, 2018. www.youtube.com/watch?v=AgdtwcLbEVg
10. Harris County Public Health. "One Year After Harvey—Eddie Scott." August 30, 2018. YouTube video. www.youtube.com/watch?v=0qIYitTV45E
11. Harris County Public Health. "One Year After Harvey—Aguero Family." August 30, 2018. YouTube video. www.youtube.com/watch?v=hnfW9KDInek
12. Kaplow JB, Layne CM, and Rolon-Arroyo B. "Evidence-Based Assessment in the Aftermath of Disasters: Towards a Best-Practice Model for Evaluating Hurricane-Exposed Youth," *Advisor*, December 2018. http://apsaclibrary.org/publications_all.php?dir=2018%20Number%204#
13. Kaplow JB, Saunders J, Angold A, et al. "Psychiatric Symptoms in Bereaved Versus Non-bereaved Youth and Young Adults: A Longitudinal, Epidemiological Study." *Journal of the American Academy of Child and Adolescent Psychiatry*, 49, 1145–1154, 2010. www.ncbi.nlm.nih.gov/pmc/articles/PMC2965565/
14. "Promoting Mental Health and Resilience Among Youths Affected by Hurricane Harvey and Its Aftermath." Robert Wood Johnson Foundation, Grant No. 75588, $1,743,726, 8/15/2018, 8/14/2020.
15. Dodd C, Hill R, Oosterhoff B, et al. "The Hurricane Exposure, Adversity, and Recovery Tool (HEART): Developing and Validating a Risk Screening Instrument for Youth Exposed to Hurricane Harvey." *Journal of Family Strengths*, 19(1), August 2019. www.researchgate.net/publication/333601296_The_Hurricane_Exposure_Adversity_and_Recovery_Tool_HEART_Developing_and_Validating_a_Risk_Screening_Instrument_for_Youth_Exposed_to_Hurricane_Harvey
16. Harvey Resiliency and Recovery Program, The Trauma and Grief Center, Texas Children's Hospital. www.texaschildrens.org/departments/trauma-and-grief-center/harvey-clinic
17. Ibid.
18. Rolon-Arroyo B, Kaplow.B, Oosterhoff B, et al. "The UCLA PTSD Reaction Index for *DSM-5* Brief Form: A Screening Tool for Trauma-Exposed Youth." *Journal of the American Academy of Child and Adolescent Psychiatry*, 59, 434–443, March 2020.
19. PENTA Consortium LLC. "Harris County Multi-Agency Coordinating Group Gap Analysis." July 2019. www.readyharris.org/Portals/43/PDFs/Harris%20County%20Gap%20Analysis%20Report%20-%20Updated%20and%20optimized.pdf?ver=2019-07-25-155525-513
20. Ibid.
21. Pabst E and Metzger L. "Illegal Air Pollution in Texas." Environment Texas Research and Policy Center. December 18, 2019. https://environmenttexas.org/sites/environment/files/reports/TX_Pollution_scrn%20%281%29.pdf
22. "Why Would Texas Officials Refuse NASA's Help After Harvey?" Editorial. *Houston Chronicle*, March 6, 2019. www.chron.com/opinion/editorials/article/Why-would-Texas-officials-refuse-NASA-s-help-13668959.php
23. Song L and Shaw A. "Independent Monitors Found Benzene Levels After Harvey Six Times Higher Than Guidelines," *ProPublica* and *The Texas Tribune*, September 14, 2017. https://projects.propublica.org/graphics/harvey-manchester
24. Air Alliance Houston. "Air Alliance Houston's Bakeyah Nelson Testifies Before Congress." February 26, 2019.
25. Ibid.

26. Byrd A. "Congress Investigates EPA for Refusing NASA's Help After Hurricane Harvey." *Colorlines*, March 7, 2019. www.colorlines.com/articles/congress-investigates-epa-refusing-nasas-help-after-hurricane-harvey

27. Nelson B. "Houston Has Fallen Behind on Fighting Air Pollution." *Houston Chronicle*, September 13, 2018. www.houstonchronicle.com/opinion/outlook/article/Houston-has-fallen-behind-on-fighting-air-13225434.php

28. Ibid.

29. Air Alliance Houston. "Rejection of NASA's Health Post-Hurricane Harvey: Statement of Bakeyah Nelson, Air Alliance Houston Executive Director, March 5, 2019." https://airalliancehouston.org/aah-statement-on-the-epa-tceqs-rejection-of-nasas-help-post-hurricane-harvey/

30. Nelson B. "Chemical Fires, Explosions Too Common in Houston." *Houston Chronical*, October 3, 2019. www.houstonchronicle.com/opinion/outlook/article/Chemical-fires-explosions-too-common-in-Houston-14487285.php

31. Fernandez M and Mervosh S. "For Some in Texas, Imelda's Heavy Rain Feels Like Harvey 2.0." *New York Times*, September 19, 2019. www.nytimes.com/2019/09/19/us/imelda-hurricane-harvey.html

Chapter 12

1. Fountain H and Popovich N. "2019 Was the Second-Hottest Year Ever, Closing Out the Warmest Decade." *New York Times*, January 15, 2020. www.nytimes.com/interactive/2020/01/15/climate/hottest-year-2019.html

2. Crimmins A, Balbus J, Gamble JL, et al. "Populations of Concern. The Impacts of Climate Change on Human Health in the United States: A Scientific Assessment." *U.S. Global Change Research Program, Climate and Health Assessment*. Chapter 9 GlobalChange.org. http://dx.doi.org/10.7930/J0R49NQX

3. Plough A. "The Impact of Climate Change on Health and Equity." *Culture of Health Blog*. Robert Wood Johnson Foundation. June 22, 2016. www.rwjf.org/content/rwjf/en/blog/2016/06/what_does_climatech.html

4. Bullard R, Gardezi M, Chennault C, et al. "Climate Change and Environmental Justice: A Conversation With Dr. Robert Bullard." *Journal of Critical Thought and Praxis*, 5(2), 2016. https://lib.dr.iastate.edu/jctp/vol5/iss2/3/.

5. Painter M and Gandhi P. "How Communities Are Promoting Health and Responding to Climate Change." Culture of Health Blog. Robert Wood Johnson Foundation. September 30, 2019. www.rwjf.org/en/blog/2019/09/how-communities-are-promoting-health-and-responding-to-climate-change.html

6. Climate and Health Program, Centers for Disease Control and Prevention. "Celebrating 10 Years." November 6, 2019. www.cdc.gov/climateandhealth/default.htm

7. U.S. Global Change Research Program. *Fourth National Climate Assessment: Volume II: Impacts, Risks, and Adaptation in the United States*. 2018. https://nca2018.globalchange.gov/

8. Climate Central. "U.S. Faces Dramatic Rise in Extreme Heat, Humidity." July 2013. http://assets.climatecentral.org/pdfs/Heat_methodology.pdf

9. Hoerner JA and Robinson N. "A Climate of Change: African-Americans, Global Warming and Just Climate Policy." Environmental Justice and Climate Change Initiative, 2008. https://urbanhabitat.org/files/climateofchange.pdf

10. Anderson M, and McMinn S. "As Rising Heat Bakes U.S. Cities, the Poor Often Feel It Most." Heat and Health in American Cities. All Things Considered, National Public Radio. September 3, 2019. www.npr.org/2019/09/03/754044732/as-rising-heat-bakes-u-s-cities-the-poor-often-feel-it-most

11. Hoffman J, Shandas V, Pendleton N. "The Effects of Historical Housing Policies on Resident Exposure to Intra-Urban Heat: A Study of 108 US Urban Areas." *Climate*, January 13, 2020. www.mdpi.com/2225-1154/8/1/12/htm

12. McKenna P. "EPA Finds Black Americans Face More Health-Threatening Air Pollution," *Inside Climate News*, March 2, 2018. www.insideclimatenews.org/news/01032018/air-pollution-data-african-american-race-health-epa-research

13. Eckert N. "How High Heat Can Impact Mental Health." Heat and Health in American Cities, All Things Considered, National Public Radio, September 4, 2019. www.npr.org/2019/09/04/757034136/how-high-heat-can-impact-mental-health

14. Centers for Disease Control and Prevention. "BRACE Framework." Climate and Health.www.cdc.gov/climateandhealth/BRACE.htm

15. Kaw Nation EPA Office. "Climate Change and Human Health: Adverse Health Effects of Extreme Precipitation Fact Sheet." www.nihb.org/docs/08142019/Brochure%20-%20Extreme%20Precipitation.pdf

16. San Francisco Department of Public Health. "San Francisco Vulnerability to the Health Impacts of Extreme Heat: A Story Map." https://arcg.is/1HK89j

17. "What's New." *Climate and Health News*. Centers for Disease Control and Prevention. Accessed on July 20, 2020. www.cdc.gov/climateandhealth/whats-new.htm

18. Pala Environmental Department. "Climate Change: Extreme Heat and Pala." Example of tip sheet produced by the Pala Environmental Department. http://ped.palatribe.com/climate-change-extreme-heat-and-pala/

19. Fillion R. "How 2019 Became the Year When the World Woke Up to the Climate Emergency." *ScienceAlert*, December 29, 2019. www.sciencealert.com/how-2019-became-the-year-when-the-world-woke-up-to-the-climate-emergency

20. Bullard RD. *The Quest for Environmental Justice: Human Rights and the Politics of Pollution*. San Francisco: Sierra Club Books, 2005.

21. Bullard RD. "Solid Waste Sites and the Black Houston Community." *Sociological Inquiry*, 53(2–3), April 1983. https://onlinelibrary.wiley.com/doi/abs/10.1111/j.1475-682X.1983.tb00037.x

22. Bullard RD. *Invisible Houston: The Black Experience in Boom and Bust*. College Station, TX: Texas A&M University Press, 1987.

23. Bullard RD. *Confronting Environmental Racism: Voices From the Grassroots*. Boston: South End Press, 1993.

24. U.S. Department of Health and Human Services, Office of Minority Health. "Asthma and African Americans." Last modified January 9, 2018. www.minorityhealth.hhs.gov/omh/browse.aspx?lvl=4&lvlid=15

25. Bullard R. "African Americans on the Frontline Fighting for Environmental Justice." Blog post, February 22, 2019. www.drrobertbullard.com/african-americans-on-the-frontline-fighting-for-environmental-justice

26. Bullard RD and Wright B. *The Wrong Complexion for Protection*. New York: New York University Press, 2012.

27. Ruth D, McCaig A, and Fike K. "Natural Disasters Widen Racial Wealth Gap." Rice University press release about a paper called "Damages Done: The Longitudinal Impacts of Natural Hazards on Wealth Inequality in the United States." August 20, 2018. http://news.rice.edu/2018/08/20/natural-disasters-widen-racial-wealth-gap-2/

28. "Mapping Life Expectancy." Robert Wood Johnson Foundation. The RWJF Commission to Build a Healthier America has embraced mapping to show how where you live creates dramatic differences in life expectancy. www.rwjf.org/en/library/articles-and-news/2015/09/city-maps.html

29. U.S. Environmental Protection Agency. *Environmental Equity: Reducing Risks for All Communities, Volume Two: Supporting Document*. Washington., June 1992. www.epa.gov/sites/production/files/2015-02/documents/reducing_risk_com_vol2.pdf

30. Huang A. "The 20th Anniversary of President Clinton's Executive Order 12898 on Environmental Justice." *Expert Blog*, February 10, 2014. www.nrdc.org/experts/albert-huang/20th-anniversary-president-clintons-executive-order-12898-environmental-justice

31. Bullard R. "Dr. Robert Bullard Named to List of World's 100 Most Influential People in Climate Policy 2019." March 28, 2019. News release. https://drrobertbullard.com/dr-robert-d-bullard-named-to-list-of-worlds-100-most-influential-people-in-climate-policy-2019/

32. Lohan T. "Dr. Robert Bullard: Lessons From 40 Years of Documenting Environmental Racism." *The Revelator*, April 17, 2019. www.therevelator.org/bullard-environmental-justice/

33. Bullard R. "Time for Whites to Stop Dumping Their Pollution on People of Color." Blog post, April 2, 2019. www.drrobertbullard.com/time-for-Whites-to-stop-dumping-their-pollution-on-people-of-color/

34. Cruz G. "Top 10 Environmental Disasters: And the Earth Cried: Love Canal." *TIME Magazine,* May 3, 2010. http://content.time.com/time/specials/packages/article/0,28804,1986457_1986501_1986441,00.html

35. Information about the Deep South Center for Environmental Justice available online. http://www.dscej.org/our-story

36. "Gulf Equity Water Corps: Students Raising Awareness about Sea Level Rise and Flooding Along the Gulf Coast." www.fluxconsole.com/files/item/211/59227/StudentsRaisingAwarenessAboutSeaLevelRisearticle.pdf

37. Deep South Center for Environmental Justice. "Taking Steps Together on Equity & Climate Change: A Report by and for New Orleanians." Climate Action Equity Report. September 2019. http://www.dscej.org/the-latest/new-orleans-residents-put-forward-climate-solutions-that-achieve-equity

38. Taylor Williams R. "Achieving Sustainability through Education and Economic Development Solutions." Poster presentation at *Sharing Knowledge* conference, Houston. Project in Duck Hill, Mississippi. 2019.

39. Robert Wood Johnson Foundation. ID 76372, $503,840: Developing a strong cadre of Intergenerational citizen leaders to advance resilience and equity in North Montgomery County, Mississippi. April 15, 2019–April 14, 2021.

40. Boyd R. "The People of the Isle de Jean Charles Are Louisiana's First Climate Refugees—but They Won't be the Last." *NRCD,* September 23, 2019. www.nrdc.org/stories/people-isle-jean-charles-are-louisianas-first-climate-refugees-they-wont-be-last

41. Robert Wood Johnson Foundation. "Global Ideas for U.S. Solutions: Cities Taking Action to Address Health, Equity, and Climate Change." March 23, 2020. www.rwjf.org/en/library/funding-opportunities/2020/global-ideas-for-us-solutions-cities-taking-action-to-address-health-equity-and-climate-change.html

42. Painter M and Gandhi P. "How Communities Are Promoting Health and Responding to Climate Change." *Culture of Health Blog.* Robert Wood Johnson Foundation. September 30, 2019. www.rwjf.org/en/blog/2019/09/how-communities-are-promoting-health-and-responding-to-climate-change.html

Spotlight

1. Information about Climate Interactive is available at www.climateinteractive.org

2. Sawin E. "The Magic of Multisolving." *Stanford Social Innovation Review,* July 16, 2018. https://ssir.org/articles/entry/the_magic_of_multisolving

3. Sawin E, McCauley S, Edberg S, et al. "Multisolving at the Intersection of Health and Climate Change: Lessons From Success Stories." Climate Interactive. January 2018. Support for this report was provided in part by the Robert Wood Johnson Foundation. www.climateinteractive.org/wp-content/uploads/2018/01/Multisolving-at-the-Intersection-of-Health-and-Climate.pdf

4. "Health Benefits Far Outweigh the Costs of Meeting Climate Change Goals." World Health Organization. December 5, 2018. www.who.int/news-room/detail/05-12-2018-health-benefits-far-outweigh-the-costs-of-meeting-climate-change-goals

Chapter 13

1. Research Ethics. "Institutional Review Boards and the Belmont Principles." Boston University School of Public Health, 2016. http://sphweb.bumc.bu.edu/otlt/MPH-Modules/EP/EP713_ResearchEthics/EP713_ResearchEthics3.html

2. American Psychological Association. "Frequently Asked Questions About Institutional Review Boards." Washington: American Psychological Association, 2020. www.apa.org/advocacy/research/defending-research/review-boards

3. Singer N. "Apple's Reach Reshapes Medical Research." *New York Times*, November 14, 2019. www.nytimes.com/2019/11/14/technology/apple-harvard-health-studies.html?smtyp=cur

4. Office for Human Research Protections. *The Belmont Report: Ethical Principles and Guidelines for the Protection of Human Subjects of Research*. Washington: U.S. Department of Health and Human Services, April 1979. www.hhs.gov/ohrp/regulations-and-policy/belmont-report/read-the-belmont-report/index.html

5. Department of Homeland Security: Science and Technology. "The Menlo Report: Ethical Principles Guiding Information and Communication Technology Research." U.S. Department of Homeland Security, August 2012. www.caida.org/publications/papers/2012/menlo_report_actual_formatted/menlo_report_actual_formatted.pdf

6. Food and Drug Administration. "Digital Health Software Precertification (Pre-Cert) Program." FDA, 2020. www.fda.gov/medical-devices/digital-health/digital-health-software-precertification-pre-cert-program

7. Pérez-Peña R and Rosenberg M. "Strava Fitness App Can Reveal Military Sites, Analysts Say." *New York Times*, January 29, 2018. www.nytimes.com/2018/01/29/world/middleeast/strava-heat-map.html

8. Ibid.

9. Holoubek S and Hibbard J. "Problem Spotlight: Algorithmic Bias and Health." Luminary Labs, 2019. www.luminary-labs.com/insight/problem-spotlight-algorithmic-bias-and-health/

10. Hamilton IA. "Why It's Totally Unsurprising That Amazon's Recruitment AI Was Biased Against Women." *Business Insider*, October 13, 2018. www.businessinsider.com/amazon-ai-biased-against-women-no-surprise-sandra-wachter-2018-10

11. Angwin J, Larson J, Mattu S, et al. "Machine Bias." *ProPublica*, May 23, 2016. www.propublica.org/article/machine-bias-risk-assessments-in-criminal-sentencing

12. Institute for the Future and Omidyar Network. *Ethical OS: A Guide to Anticipating the Future Impact of Today's Technology—Or: How Not to Regret the Things You Will Build*. Palo Alto, CA: Institute for the Future and Redwood City, CA, and Omidyar Network, 2018. https://ethicalos.org/

13. *Digital Health Decision-Making Framework and Checklist Designed for Researchers*. San Diego: ReCODE Health, 2020. https://recode.health/tools/

14. UC San Diego, Research Center for Optimal Digital Ethics Health. "ReCODE Health," 2019. https://recode.health/

15. UC San Diego, Research Center for Optimal Digital Ethics in Health. "The CORE Platform," 2019. http://thecore-platform.ucsd.edu/

16. Hill D. *Project HealthDesign: Rethinking the Power and Potential of Personal Health Records*. Princeton, NJ: Robert Wood Johnson Foundation, 2015. www.rwjf.org/en/library/research/2010/10/project-healthdesign--rethinking-the-power-and-potential-of-pers.html

17. Tarini P. Engaging Patients in Research. *Culture of Health Blog*. Robert Wood Johnson Foundation. 2013. www.rwjf.org/en/blog/2013/11/engaging_patientsin.html

18. Robert Wood Johnson Foundation. "Designing, Building, and Testing a Web-Based Prototype to Foster the Ethical Design and Review of Health Research." Grant ID 27876 to University of California, San Diego, School of Medicine. November 2015 through April 2019.

19. Ferryman K and Pitcan M. "What Is Precision Medicine? Contemporary Issues and Concerns Primer." Data & Society, 2018. https://datasociety.net/pubs/pm/DataandSociety_What_Is_Precision_Medicine_Primer_2018.pdf

Spotlight

1. Information about the HUMAN Project available at www.kavlifoundation.org/kavli-human-project

Chapter 14

1. Information about the Value of Health tool is available at https://altarum.org/projects/measuring-value-health
2. A detailed description of the framework is available in Miller G, Roehrig C, and Russo P. "A Framework for Assessing the Value of Investments in Nonclinical Prevention." *Preventing Chronic Disease, 12*, December 10, 2015. www.cdc.gov/pcd/issues/2015/15_0363.htm.
3. Pew Charitable Trusts. "10 Policies to Prevent and Respond to Childhood Lead Exposure." A report from the Health Impact Project of the Pew Charitable Trusts. Philadelphia, PA. August 30, 2017. www.pewtrusts.org/en/research-and-analysis/reports/2017/08/10-policies-to-prevent-and-respond-to-childhood-lead-exposure
4. The Value of Lead Prevention tool is available at http://valueofleadprevention.org
5. Information about Collaborative Approach to Public Good Investment (CAPGI) is available at https://capgi.gmu.edu/index.php/intro-to-capgi-for-strangers/
6. Nichols LM and Taylor LA. "Social Determinants as Public Goods: A New Approach to Financing Key Investments in Healthy Communities." *Health Affairs, 37*(8), August 2018. www.healthaffairs.org/doi/full/10.1377/hlthaff.2018.0039
7. Cannon JS, Kilburn MR, Karoly LA, et al. "Investing Early: Taking Stock of Outcomes and Economic Returns From Early Childhood Programs." RAND Corporation, 2017. www.rand.org/pubs/research_reports/RR1993.html
8. Karoly LA, Kilburn MR, and Cannon JS. *Early Childhood Interventions: Proven Results, Future Promise.* MG-341. Santa Monica, Calif.: RAND Corporation, 2005. www.rand.org/pubs/monographs/MG341.html
9. U.S. Centers for Medicare & Medicaid Services. "April 2020 Medicaid & CHIP Enrollment Data Highlights." Last updated July 23, 2020. www.medicaid.gov/medicaid/program-information/medicaid-and-chip-enrollment-data/report-highlights/index.html
10. U.S. Centers for Medicare & Medicaid Services. "NHE Fact Sheet." National Health Expenditure Data. March 24, 2020. www.cms.gov/research-statistics-data-and-systems/statistics-trends-and-reports/nationalhealthexpenddata/nhe-fact-sheet.html
11. Hinton E, Rudowitz R, Diaz M, et al. "10 Things to Know About Medicaid Managed Care." Kaiser Family Foundation, September 6, 2019. www.kff.org/medicaid/issue-brief/10-things-to-know-about-medicaid-managed-care/
12. Livingston S. "Social Determinants Are Core of North Carolina's Medicaid Overhaul." *Modern Healthcare*, August 3, 2018. www.modernhealthcare.com/article/20180803/TRANSFORMATION01/180809944/social-determinants-are-core-of-north-carolina-s-medicaid-overhaul.

Conclusion

1. McGinnis M, Williams-Russo P, and Knickman J. "The Case for More Active Policy Attention to Health Promotion." *Health Affairs* (Millwood), *21*, 78–93, 2002. www.healthaffairs.org/doi/full/10.1377/hlthaff.21.2.78
2. Schroeder S. "We Can Do Better—Improving the Health of the American People." *New England Journal of Medicine, 357*, 1221–1228, 2007. www.nejm.org/doi/full/10.1056/nejmsa073350
3. Krieger N. "Health Equity and the Fallacy of Treating Causes of Population Health as If They Sum to 100%." *American Journal of Public Health,107*(4), 541–549, April 2017. www.ncbi.nlm.nih.gov/pmc/articles/PMC5343713

INDEX

For the benefit of digital users, indexed terms that span two pages (e.g., 52–53) may, on occasion, appear on only one of those pages.

CULTURE OF HEALTH ACTION FRAMEWORK

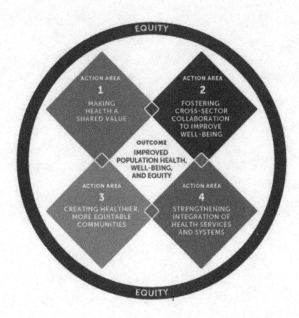